PHLEBOTOMY

FOR HEALTH CARE PERSONNEL

PHLEBOTOMY

FOR HEALTH CARE PERSONNEL

Second Edition

Kathryn A. Booth, RN-BSN, MS, RMA, RPT

*Total Care Programming
Palm Coast, Florida*

**Antonio C. Wallace, BS-HCM, CPT,
CAHI, CICS, MSS, FSS, NCMA**

*MDEC (Medical/Dental & Educational
Consulting Co.) Atlanta, Georgia*

Debbie T. Fitzgerald, RN, BSN, MS, ABD

*McGraw-Hill Higher Education
Burr Ridge, IL*

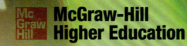

**McGraw-Hill
Higher Education**

Boston   Burr Ridge, IL   Dubuque, IA   New York   San Francisco   St. Louis
Bangkok   Bogotá   Caracas   Kuala Lumpur   Lisbon   London   Madrid   Mexico City
Milan   Montreal   New Delhi   Santiago   Seoul   Singapore   Sydney   Taipei   Toronto

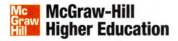

McGraw-Hill
Higher Education

PHLEBOTOMY FOR HEALTH CARE PERSONNEL, SECOND EDITION

Published by McGraw-Hill, a business unit of The McGraw-Hill Companies, Inc., 1221 Avenue of the Americas, New York, NY, 10020. Copyright © 2009, 2002 by The McGraw-Hill Companies, Inc. All rights reserved. No part of this publication may be reproduced or distributed in any form or by any means, or stored in a database or retrieval system, without the prior written consent of The McGraw-Hill Companies, Inc., including, but not limited to, in any network or other electronic storage or transmission, or broadcast for distance learning.

Some ancillaries, including electronic and print components, may not be available to customers outside the United States.

This book is printed on acid-free paper.

5 6 7 8 9 0 WDQ/WDQ 12 11 10

ISBN 978-0-07-351097-2

MHID 0-07-351097-1

Vice President/Editor in Chief: *Elizabeth Haefele*
Vice President/Director of Marketing: *John E. Biernat*
Sponsoring editor: *Debbie Fitzgerald*
Developmental editor: *Connie Kuhl*
Executive marketing manager: *Roxan Kinsey*
Lead media producer: *Damian Moshak*
Media producer: *Ben Curless*
Director, Editing/Design/Production: *Jess Ann Kosic*
Project manager: *Jean R. Starr*
Production supervisor: *Janean A. Utley*
Designer: *Srdjan Savanovic*

Photo research coordinator: *Lori Hancock*
Photo researcher: *LouAnn Wilson*
Media project manager: *Mark Dierker*
Cover/interior design: *Studio Montage*
Typeface: *10.5/13 Melior*
Compositor: *ICC Macmillan Inc.*
Printer: *Worldcolor, Dubuque*
Cover credit: © David Buffington/Getty Images
Credits: The credits section for this book begins on page 248 and is considered an extension of the copyright page.

Library of Congress Cataloging-in-Publication Data

Booth, Kathryn (Kathryn A.)
    Phlebotomy for health care personnel / Kathryn A. Booth, Antonio A. Wallace, Debbie T. Fitzgerald.
        p. ; cm.
    Includes index.
    Rev. ed. of: Glencoe phlebotomy for health care personnel / Debbie T. Fitzgerald, Linda A. Dezern. c2002.
        ISBN-13: 978-0-07-351097-2 (alk. paper)
        ISBN-10: 0-07-351097-1 (alk. paper)
        1. Phlebotomy—Handbooks, manuals, etc. I. Wallace, Antonio. II. Fitzgerald, Debbie T., 1963- III. Fitzgerald, Debbie T., 1963- Glencoe phlebotomy for health care personnel. IV. Title.
    [DNLM: 1. Phlebotomy—methods—Handbooks. 2. Blood Circulation—Handbooks. QY 39 B725p 2009]
    RB45.15.F586 2009
    616.07'561—dc22

                                                                                2007043017

The Internet addresses listed in the text were accurate at the time of publication. The inclusion of a Web site does not indicate an endorsement by the authors or McGraw-Hill, and McGraw-Hill does not guarantee the accuracy of the information presented at these sites.

WARNING NOTICE: The clinical procedures, medicines, dosages, and other matters described in this publication are based upon research of current literature and consultation with knowledgeable persons in the field. The procedures and matters described in this text reflect currently accepted clinical practice. However, this information cannot and should not be relied upon as necessarily applicable to a given individual's case. Accordingly, each person must be separately diagnosed to discern the patient's unique circumstances. Likewise, the manufacturer's package insert for current drug product information should be consulted before administering any drug. Publisher disclaims all liability for any inaccuracies, omissions, misuse, or misunderstanding of the information contained in this publication. Publisher cautions that this publication is not intended as a substitute for the professional judgment of trained medical personnel.

www.mhhe.com

Dedication

To the users of this program, congratulations on your selection of an essential career in health care. The skills and abilities learned in this program will provide you a lifetime of employment in a much needed profession. To my family, all of whom have made this a great year, and especially to TJ for his endless spirit and good heart.

Kathryn Booth

To all the health care providers who use this textbook, congratulations on your chosen career path. It is a privilege to assist you with obtaining valuable knowledge and skills that will guide you through the learning phase of this journey. To my family and friends, who have stood by me during this journey, especially my mother, Eva Wallace, and my sisters, Aletha, Tressa, Juanita, Sharon, and Rena, my friends, Lonnie, Anita, Derek, Jay, Donald, Jerry, and Kenyan, Marilyn and Dr. Tonjie Scott. I truly appreciate the love and support.

Antonio Wallace

To my family and friends for their continued love and support. A special acknowledgment to the many students who have kept me in their lives long after completing courses I've taught. It has been wonderful to learn of your successes!

Debbie Fitzgerald

About the Authors

Kathryn A. Booth, RN, BSN, MS, RMA, is a full-time author, educator, and consultant for Total Care Programming, a multimedia software development company. Her background includes a bachelor's degree in nursing and a master's degree in education. Her twenty-eight years of teaching, nursing, and health care work experience spans five states. She has authored and developed multimedia software and health care textbooks and educational materials for McGraw Hill Higher Education; Total Care Programming; Glencoe/McGraw-Hill; Mosby Lifeline; and Lippincott, Williams, and Wilkins. Mrs. Booth has presented at numerous state, corporate, and national conventions since 1994. Her current focus is to develop up-to-date, dynamic health care education materials to assist educators and promote the health care profession. To remain current, Kathy has most recently worked as a part-time LPN instructor and a practicing medical assistant, and she has just completed her RMA and RPT certification.

Antonio Wallace, CPT, CAHI, CICS, MSS, FSS, NCMA, owner and operator of MDEC, a Medical/Dental & Educational Consulting Company located in Atlanta, Georgia, which focuses on providing quality training for schools, physician and dental offices to include hospitals and other entities that need assistance with raising the bar in their organizations and institutions. His background includes a bachelor's degree in health care management. He is aggressively pursuing a master's degree. He has been in the education-health care industry for more than twenty years, serving in such positions as Director of Education, Interim School Director, Medical Program Chair/Director, Externship Director, Allied Health Instructor, Basic Sciences to include Anatomy and Physiology Instructor, Phlebotomy Instructor, Medical Billing and Coding Instructor, Clinical Medical Instructor, EKG Instructor, Medical Office Operations Manager, Clinic Manager, Medical Office Manager, just to name a few. He currently holds the following credentials Certified Phlebotomy Technician, Certified Allied Health Instructor, Certified Insurance and Coding Specialist, Medical Services Specialist, Financial Services Specialist, National Certified Medical Assistant, Certified EKG Specialist. He has also written medical based programs for some local proprietary schools and two-year colleges in the Atlanta, Georgia area. He is originally from Texas, but has lived in Georgia for almost twenty years.

Debbie Fitzgerald, RN, BSN, MS, ABD, Senior Sponsoring Editor for McGraw-Hill Higher Education, received her bachelor's degree in nursing and master's degree in nursing education. Mrs. Fitzgerald is currently completing her dissertation for the doctor of philosophy degree in organizational leadership with a cognate in education. She has over ten years teaching experience with LPN and Medical Assisting Education and served as the Program Leader of Health Occupations. She has served as co-author, contributing author, and consultant. Mrs. Fitzgerald has presented at numerous state and national workshops and conventions on educational topics to improve student engagement.

Brief Contents

Contents

Preface

The field of health care is an ever-changing and growing place. Whether this is your first choice career or you are cross-training, the demand for qualified phlebotomists is expanding. Flexibility is key to obtaining, maintaining, and improving your health career. The concept of cross-training, or multiskilling, although not a new one, has become the expected rather than the exception. Cross-training allows you to be able to function in a variety of workplace settings doing diverse tasks. The fact that you are currently reading this book means that you are willing to acquire new skills or specialize the skills you already possess. This willingness translates into your enhanced value, job security, marketability, and mobility.

This second edition of *Phlebotomy for Health Care Personnel* was designed not just for classroom but also independent and distance learning. Checkpoint questions and Student CD exercises have been added to make the learning process interactive and to promote increased comprehension. The variety of materials included with the program provides for multiple learning styles and ensures that you will be a success.

The text/workbook/CD is divided into seven chapters:

- Chapter 1, Introduction to Phlebotomy, helps you gain a better understanding of exactly what phlebotomy involves and what it takes to become a phlebotomist. History, roles and responsibilities, safety and infection control, and legal and ethical issues are included in this chapter.

- Chapter 2, Blood Circulation, Function, and Composition, includes basic and essential information about the blood and circulatory system. This knowledge is necessary to understand the phlebotomy procedure and various tests that are performed on blood.

- Chapter 3, Equipment for Specimen Collection, details the types of equipment you will use during the practice of phlebotomy. Lots of figures have been included to ensure you are familiar with the equipment. An emphasis upon the need for safety equipment is stressed.

- Chapter 4, Performing Venipuncture and Dermal Puncture, includes the step-by-step process for both venipuncture and dermal puncture. Detailed descriptions, possible circumstances that can occur during the process, photographs, and interactive exercises on the Student CD prepare you to perform your first venipuncture or dermal puncture.

- Chapter 5, Specimen Handling and Processing, identifies the requirements for special handling and/or processing of specimens before, during, and after the collection. Specific collection processes, urine specimens, blood smears, centrifuge operation, and point-of-care and waived testing are also included in this chapter.

- Chapter 6, Special Phlebotomy Procedures, includes timed specimens; glucose testing; bleeding time and platelet function; blood donation and therapeutic collection; blood alcohol, toxicology, and forensic specimens; therapeutic drug monitoring; and alternative collection sites.

- Chapter 7, Practicing Phlebotomy, includes what you need to know to enter the field and practice as a phlebotomist. Certification, continuing education, quality assurance, quality control, factors that affect laboratory values, specimen rejection, and risk management are all addressed.

Features of the Text/Workbook/CD

Key Terms, Glossary, and Audio Glossary   Key terms are identified at the beginning of each chapter. These terms are in **bold** type within the chapter and are defined both in the chapter and in the glossary at the end of the book. Open the Student CD to hear the pronunciation of each key term, and practice learning the term with the Key Term Concentration game.

Checkpoint Questions   At the end of each main heading in the chapter are short-answer Checkpoint Questions. Answer these questions to make sure you have learned the basic concepts presented.

CD activities   After you have finished the Checkpoint Questions, you are sent to the interactive Student CD activity to further your review and practice of the concepts presented in each section. Be sure to complete the activities on the CD before you continue to the next section.

Troubleshooting   The Troubleshooting feature identifies problems and situations that may arise when you are caring for patients or performing a procedure. At the end of this feature, you are asked a question to answer in your own words.

Safety and Infection Control   You are responsible for providing safe care and preventing the spread of infection. This feature presents tips and techniques to help you practice these important skills relative to phlebotomy.

Patient Education and Communication   Patient interaction and education and intrateam communication are integral parts of health care. As part of your daily duties, you must communicate effectively both orally and in writing, and you must provide patient education. Use this feature to learn ways to perform these tasks.

HIPAA, Law, and Ethics   When working in health care, you must be conscious of the regulations of HIPAA (Health Insurance Portability and Accountability Act) and understand your legal responsibilities and the implications of your actions. You must perform duties within established ethical practices. This feature helps you gain insight into how HIPAA, law, and ethics relate to the performance of your duties.

Chapter Summary and Review   Once you have completed each chapter, take time to read the summary and complete the chapter review questions, which are presented in a variety of formats. These questions help you understand the content presented in each chapter.

Get Connected and the Online Learning Center   The Get Connected activity directs you to the Online Learning Center (OLC) that accompanies the text/workbook. The OLC provides links for you to complete research and activities relative to the information presented in the chapter. You will also find other review activities and materials on the OLC to assist you in learning phlebotomy.

Chapter Test   Open the Student CD to take a final test of your knowledge relative to each chapter. Review the material again with the Spin the Wheel game and then take the chapter test. You can print or e-mail your score to your instructor.

Instructor's Manual and Instructor CD

Look to the Instructor's Manual and the Instructor CD for multiple resources to use while teaching *Phlebotomy for Health Care Personnel.* PowerPoint presentations for each chapter have Apply Your Knowledge questions at the end of each section and can be used for classroom presentation and discussion. An EZ-Test test bank that contains a variety of questions with graphics allows you to simply and easily create your own final or chapter exam. Also available are suggested classroom activities that will increase the interest level and comprehension of the text/workbook/CD material. Anticipatory set activities for each chapter help stimulate and enhance student learning as you begin each new topic. Curriculum suggestions provide information on how to use the materials based on your course length and depth. All media on the Student CD are conveniently provided on the Instructor CD for classroom presentations.

Acknowledgments

Kathryn Booth

Thanks to the graduating Medical Assistant students at Daytona Beach Community College under the direction of Suzanne Fielding and Mike McCumber. They provided us a location for photography and videotaping for the textbook and software program. Suzanne Fielding gets special thanks for making all the arrangements and providing technical expertise throughout the photography. Also many thanks go to Leesa Whicker and her Medical Assistant students at Central Piedmont Community College in Charlotte, NC, for their time during the video and photography session at their facility.

Antonio Wallace

Thanks to Dr. Marie Jarrett at Georgia Perimeter College, Shirley Webb at Javelin Technical Training Center, Lisa McGreer Staples at Advanced Career Training, Hannah Leonard Hinds at Westwood College, among others who allowed me to monitor their classes and obtain valuable information conducive to preparing this textbook for phlebotomy professionals.

Debbie Fitzgerald

Thanks to the awesome editorial team at McGraw-Hill Higher Education for their tireless efforts and continued excellence.

Consultants

Jennifer Childers, MS, PA-C
Assistant Professor of Physician Assistant Studies
Alderson Broaddus College Philippi, WV

Cheri Goretti, MA, MT(ASCP), CMA
Quinebaug Valley Community College
Danielson, CT

Lynn M. Peterson, M.Ed., I(ASCP) SI, QCYM
Carroll College
Waukesha, WI

Cynthia T. Vincent, MMS, PA-C
Coordinator, Physician Assistant Master's Degree Completion Program
Alderson Broaddus College Philippi, WV

Mollie Weaver, BSMT (ASCP)
South Arkansas Community College
El Dorado, AR

Reviewer Acknowledgments

Dr. Joseph H. Balatbat
Vice President of Academics
Sanford Brown Institute–New York City
New York, NY

Richard T. Boan, PhD
Midlands Technical College
Columbia, SC

Lou M. Brown
Wayne Community College
Goldsboro, NC

Patricia A. Chappell
Camden County College
Blackwood, NJ

Shelley S. Cheney, AS, CMA
High-Tech Institute
Las Vegas, NV

Pamela Fleming
Quinsigamond Community College
Worcester, MA

Kathleen L. Garza
Hocking College
Nelsonville, OH

Cheri Goretti, MA, MT(ASCP),
    CMA
Quinebaug Valley Community
    College
Danielson, CT

Sabrina Judilla-Cruz, MD
Sanford Brown Institute–NYC
New York, NY

Karen A. Kittle
Oakland Community College
Waterford, MI

Tracie Lichfield
Phlebotomy Learning Center
Salt Lake City, UT

Jeanne R. Phelps
Wake Technical Community College
Raleigh, NC

Nadia Rajsz, Assistant Professor
Orange County Community College
Middleton, NY

Jan C. Rogers
Morrisville State College
Morrisville, NY

Danielle Schortzmann Wilken
Goodwin College
East Hartford, CT

Sharon T. Scott
Ivy Tech Community College
    of Indiana–Northwest
Gary, IN

Rita Stoffel
Red Rocks Community College
Lakewood, CO

Mollie Weaver, BSMT(ASCP)
South Arkansas Community College
El Dorado, AR

Em M. Piji Zieber
Lethbridge Community College
Lethbridge, Canada

Guided Tour

Features to Help You Study and Learn

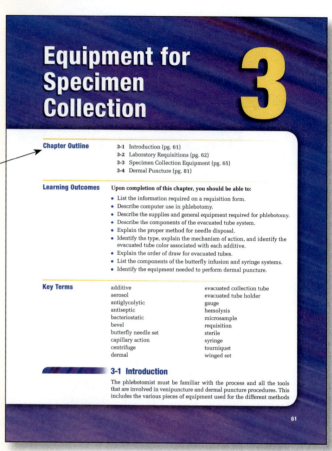

Chapter Outlines, Learning Outcomes, Key Terms, and an Introduction begin each chapter to introduce you to the chapter and help prepare you for the information that will be presented.

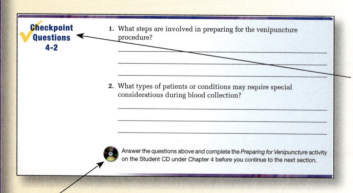

Checkpoint Questions are provided at the end of each section in the chapter to help you understand the information you just read.

CD-ROM references direct you to the interactive CD activity to further your review and practice the concepts presented in each section.

Troubleshooting exercises identify problems and situations that may arise on the job. You may be asked to answer a question about the situation.

Troubleshooting — **Providing Customer Service**

The patients you draw blood from are your customers. Having patients is what provides you a job, so your patients/customers should be satisfied with your service. Customer service involves providing customer satisfaction through professionalism, positive communication, and an attitude that promotes resolution to problems when they occur.

Question: You are working alone in a busy laboratory because two other phlebotomists have called in sick. The laboratory waiting area is crowded. You expect another phlebotomist to arrive in about 20 minutes. What could you do to promote positive customer service?

_____

_____

_____

Patient Education & Communication — **Computers in the Laboratory**

In many health care facilities, when a laboratory test is ordered it is entered in a computer at the patient care station or even by the physician in his office. The computer in the laboratory receives the order and prints the requisition for the phlebotomist to take to the patient (see Figure 3-2). Very specialized "laboratory information systems" are also found in clinical laboratory facilities that connect to the laboratory analyzers and remote locations, plus provide security for patient data in order to comply with HIPAA. Essentially, in these interconnected systems all patient data, orders, results, and patient charges are kept in one system.

Patient Education & Communication boxes give you helpful information communicating effectively—both orally and written—with patients.

Safety and Infection Control boxes present tips and techniques for you to apply on the job.

Safety and Infection Control — **Isolation Precaution Equipment**

Follow the guidelines for isolation precautions when entering a patient's room. If you are not certain what personal protective equipment (PPE) to wear, such as gowns, gloves, or mask, consult with the licensed practitioner caring for the patient, such as a nurse. *Never* take a tray of phlebotomy equipment into an isolation room. Take only the equipment needed for the particular draw. If you need additional equipment, you must remove all PPE before leaving the room, collect the needed supplies, then don new PPE before re-entering the room. Only the equipment to be used should be taken in, and only the tubes and the phlebotomist should leave the room. Any unused equipment or supplies must be left in the room.

HIPAA, Law & Ethics — **Confidentiality**

The phlebotomist may be privy to laboratory results. If you disclose results of any laboratory test, you will have breached patient confidentiality and may be subject to disciplinary or legal action or even a monetary fine.

HIPAA, Law & Ethics boxes help you gain insight into necessary information related to the performance of your duties.

Key points in the **Chapter Summaries** help you review what was just learned.

Chapter Summary

- Patients must be properly identified for the blood collection procedure, including their name and another form identifier such as their birth date or medical record number. If one letter or number is different in either identifier, the blood should not be drawn unless proper identification is obtained.
- Prepare patients for blood collection by explaining the procedure, letting them know they can expect to experience pain from the needlestick. Position them in a supported seated or lying position.
- Tourniquets slow the blood to the site but if left on more than one minute can cause pain to the patient and hemoconcentration of the blood specimen.
- The venipuncture and dermal puncture sites are selected based upon their location and appearance. Venipuncture is typically performed in the

"I think this is an excellent text. I would feel very confident teaching phlebotomy using this text because it presents information in a logical and comprehensive way. Despite the vast knowledge base required for phlebotomy, this text manages to focus on what is important and not get lost in the minutia." Em M. Pijl Zieber, Lethbridge Community College, Alberta Canada

Chapter Reviews consist of various methods of quizzing you. True/False, Multiple Choice, Matching, and Critical Thinking questions appeal to all types of learners.

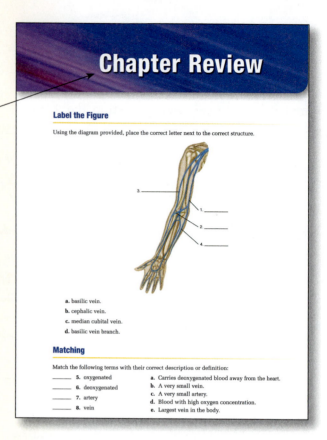

Chapter Review

Label the Figure

Using the diagram provided, place the correct letter next to the correct structure.

a. basilic vein.

b. cephalic vein.

c. median cubital vein.

d. basilic vein branch.

Matching

Match the following terms with their correct description or definition:

_____ **5.** oxygenated

_____ **6.** deoxygenated

_____ **7.** artery

_____ **8.** vein

a. Carries deoxygenated blood away from the heart.

b. A very small vein.

c. A very small artery.

d. Blood with high oxygen concentration.

e. Largest vein in the body.

Using the Student CD

Now that you have completed the material in the chapter text, return to the Student CD and complete any chapter activities you have not yet done. Practice your terminology with the "Key Term Concentration" game. Review the chapter material with the "Spin the Wheel" game. Take the final chapter test and complete the troubleshooting question. E-mail or print your results to document your proficiency for this chapter.

At the end of each chapter, you will be directed to visit the **Internet and the student CD** to experience more interactive activities about the information you just learned.

"The book and CD is very student friendly and reinforces how a person learns by reading the textbook, then answering the questions at the end of each chapter and on the CD ROM." Kathleen Garza, Hocking College, Nelsonville, OH

Introduction to Phlebotomy

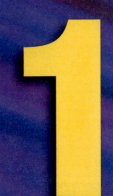

Chapter Outline

Learning Outcomes

Upon completion of this chapter, you should be able to:

- Describe the evolution of phlebotomy.
- Describe the roles and responsibilities of the phlebotomist.
- Discuss professionalism, public image, and customer service as they relate to the phlebotomist.
- Identify the various settings where phlebotomists are employed.
- List the regulating agencies for phlebotomy.
- Identify safety and infection control practices related to phlebotomy.
- Describe HIPAA, law, and ethics related to phlebotomy.

Key Terms

aseptic
capillary
Centers for Disease Control and Prevention (CDC)
chain of infection
chemistry
Clinical Laboratory Improvement Amendment (CLIA'88)
Clinical and Laboratory Standards Institute (CLSI)
confidentiality
dermal puncture
ethics
Health Insurance Portability and Accountability Act (HIPAA)

hematology
hepatitis
histology
human immunodeficiency virus (HIV)
immunology
isolation precautions
microbiology
microcollection
microsurgery
microtechnique
negligence
nosocomial infection
Occupational Safety and Health Administration (OSHA)

Patient's Bill of Rights
personal protective equipment
    (PPE)
phlebotomist
phlebotomy
point-of-care testing (POCT)
professionalism

reference laboratory
serology
Standard Precautions
toxicology
urinalysis
venipuncture

1-1 Introduction

Phlebotomy simply means to cut into a vein. The term comes from *phlebos,* Greek for "vein" and *tome,* "to cut." This invasive procedure (procedure that invades the body through cutting or puncture) is performed by professionals known as phlebotomists. Phlebotomists must demonstrate mastery of the principles and techniques established by the **Clinical and Laboratory Standards Institute (CLSI),** formerly known as the National Committee for Clinical Laboratory Standards (NCCLS).

The primary role of a **phlebotomist** is to obtain blood specimens for diagnostic testing, either by **venipuncture** (puncturing the vein) or **dermal puncture** (puncturing the skin). Another role of the phlebotomist is to remove blood from donors for blood transfusions, or from patients with a condition called polycythemia (overproduction of red blood cells), in which blood must be removed to decrease the viscosity (thickness) of the blood. Phlebotomists are also responsible for collecting and properly packaging urine specimens, accepting incoming specimens (blood and body fluids, etc.), and routing specimens to the proper departments to be tested and analyzed.

**Checkpoint
Question
1-1**

1. Name at least two functions of a phlebotomist.

_____

_____

_____

1-2 History of Phlebotomy

The process of removing blood from the veins is believed to date back as far as 1400 B.C., where an Egyptian tomb painting shows a leech being applied to the skin of a sick person. In the early 1800s leeches were in demand for the procedure known as bloodletting. Leech farms were unable to keep up with the demands for medicinal leeches because bloodletting procedures were so popular.

Bloodletting was thought to rid the body of impurities and evil spirits or, as in the time of Hippocrates, simply to return the body to a balanced state. During the 1800s anyone claiming medical training could perform bloodletting, and barbers most typically performed this procedure. A loss of approximately 10 milliliters (about two teaspoons) was standard. However, it was not uncommon for an excessive amount of blood to be withdrawn during these procedures. In fact, the untimely death of the first United States president, George Washington, was thought to be the result of excessive bloodletting in an attempt to treat a throat infection. Interestingly, the use of leeches has resurfaced with a new purpose: to remove blood that has collected at newly transplanted tissue sites, in order to decrease the swelling following **microsurgery.** Microsurgery involves reconstruction of small tissue structures.

Bloodletting also used a process called "venesection," in which the vein was pierced with a sharp object to drain blood. The lancet, a very sharp instrument used for cutting the vein, was the most popular medical instrument of that time. This method was used because it was thought to have removed or eliminated any unwanted diseases from the body, and it was also used as a way to reduce a fever. It is important to note that **aseptic,** or microorganism-free, practices were unknown during that time, so the same lancet was used on several patients without any cleansing. Another method used for bloodletting at that same time was called "cupping." This method produced a vacuum effect by pulling blood to the capillaries under a heated glass cup, which was placed on the patient's back to allow the blood to flow more. Then a spring-loaded box containing multiple blades made slices or piercings into the skin to produce bleeding. The procedure typically produced scar tissue.

During the late 1980s and early 1990s, the phlebotomy profession emerged as a result of technology and expansions of laboratory function. Initially, only medical technologists and medical technicians were responsible for collecting blood specimens, but as technology and the health care industry underwent rapid changes in the past few decades, specimen collection was delegated to other groups of trained professionals, including the phlebotomist.

✓ **Checkpoint Question 1-2**

1. Name various reasons bloodletting (early phlebotomy) was performed?

_____

_____

_____

_____

Answer the question above and complete the *History of Phlebotomy* activity on the Student CD under Chapter 1 before you continue to the next section.

1-3 Roles and Responsibilities of the Phlebotomist

The phlebotomist is a valuable member of the health care team and is responsible for the collection, processing, and transport of blood specimens to the laboratory. Entry into phlebotomy training programs usually requires

TABLE 1-1   **Duties and Responsibilities of the Phlebotomist**

- Demonstrate professional attire, attitude, and communications
- Know facility's policies and procedures
- Properly identify patients
- Collect both venous and capillary blood specimens
- Select the appropriate and accurate specimen container for the specified tests
- Properly label, handle, and transport specimens following departmental policies
- Sort specimens received and process specimens for delivery to laboratory departments
- Perform computer operations and/or update log sheets where required
- Perform point-of-care testing and quality control check
- Observe all safety regulations

a high school diploma or its equivalent. Training programs are typically offered at hospitals, technical and private schools, and community colleges, or through continuing education courses. The course can vary from a few weeks to a few months in length, depending on the program. Several members of the health care team may be trained to perform phlebotomy, such as physicians, nurses, medical assistants, paramedics, and patient care assistants. Just as the role of these health care team members may include phlebotomy, a phlebotomist may be responsible for performing a variety of other duties. These may include transporting other specimens—such as arterial blood, urine, sputum, and tissue—to the laboratory for testing. The phlebotomist may also be responsible for performing **point-of-care testing (POCT),** such as blood glucose monitoring. Point-of-care testing is performed at the patient's bedside or a work area using portable instruments. In addition, phlebotomists perform quality control testing and various clinical and clerical duties. Table 1-1 above summarizes the essential duties and responsibilities of the phlebotomist.

Patient Identification

Prior to any patient procedure, proper identification of the patient is a crucial aspect of patient safety and a top priority. The National Patient Safety Goals established by the Joint Commission on Accreditation of Healthcare Organizations (JCAHO) recommends the use of at least two patient identifiers, not including the room number, before blood samples are obtained. As discussed later in this chapter, JCAHO is the organization that sets standards for patient care in health care facilities. To follow the National Patient Safety Goals and thus prevent an error, the phlebotomist must carefully identify every patient.

Upon entering the patient area, the phlebotomist must check the patient identification. In acute care settings, patients will have an armband or identification label bearing the patient's first and last name, hospital number, date of birth, and physician's name.

Proper identification of the patient is a three-step process (see Figure 1-1). First ask the patient to state his or her name and date of birth. (See Figure 1-2.) Be sure that you do not call the patient by name prior to this, because patients with altered mental states may simply repeat the name they hear. Next, compare the name on the test requisition form/slip to the

Figure 1-1 Follow a three-step process for correct patient identification.

Three-step process to correct patient identification

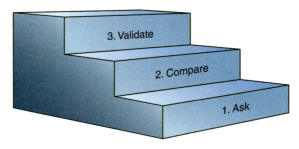

Figure 1-2 Have the patient identify himself by stating his full name and date of birth.

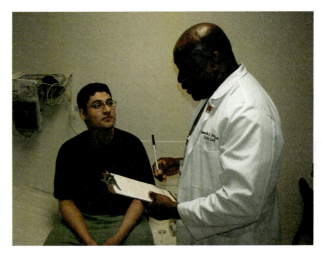

patient's response (see Figure 1-3). Finally, validate patient identification by checking the medical record number, patient armband, or some other form of identification such as a driver's license.

If this three-step process is followed, correct patient identification can be established, thereby eliminating errors. The presence of doubt at any point during the three-step check calls for further investigation of the patient's identity. If the patient is unable to state his or her name, find another source such as the nurse or a family member, depending on the setting, to state the name for you. In a hospital setting, all patients must wear an identification bracelet. Most hospital policies require that a patient have an armband in order for any procedure to be done, including phlebotomy. All laboratory specimens require a physician's order; therefore a requisition form will be available for specimens you are to collect. Remember that all specimens require proper collection, handling, labeling, and transportation to the laboratory for testing.

Specimen Collection and Handling

Physician orders for laboratory specimens will indicate the type of specimen and time of collection. Some specimens are ordered as "stat," which means they must be collected and transported immediately. Other specimens may be referred to as routine, and collection times are determined by the facility. Special laboratory tests require specific times for collection, and these are referred to as timed tests, which will be discussed in Chapter 6.

Figure 1-3 Compare the information from the laboratory requisition slip with the patient identifiers.

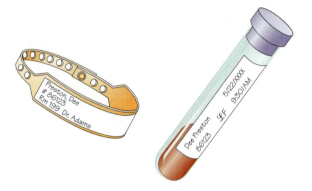

	HARBOR HOSPITAL Department of Laboratory Medicine			DATE REQUESTED 5/22/XXXX	TIME REQUESTED 9:15/AM
TEST REQUEST SLIP	TEST	RESULT	PERFORMED BY	DATE COLLECTED _____	TIME COLLECTED _____
	CBC			NAME _Dee Preston_	
				ADDRESS _99 College Blvd._ _Happy, VA_	
				PATIENT ROOM NO. _199_	BED NO. _3_
				AGE _35_ SEX _M_	HOSPITAL I.D. NO. _86123_
				PHYSICIAN _Dr. Adams_	
				TODAY ☐ ROUTINE ☒	
				EMERGENCY ☐ SIGNED	

Blood specimens provide important information that assists with the diagnosing, monitoring, and treatment of patients. The two most commonly used methods today for the collection of blood specimens are venipuncture and dermal puncture (also called a **microtechnique** or **microcollection;** see Table 1-2). Venipuncture involves the insertion of a sharp object (typically a sterile hollow core needle) into a vein to allow blood to flow into a syringe or vacuum tube. Dermal puncture requires the use of a lancet or other puncture device to prick the skin, usually the finger, for the removal of a much smaller specimen of **capillary** blood. Other sites for dermal puncture include the heel (used for infants) and earlobe. The phlebotomist must perform these tasks with confidence and expertise to ensure patient comfort. Skill is required and must be obtained through practice and experience.

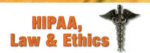

HIPAA, Law & Ethics

Patient Identification

In addition to asking the patient to state his or her name and birth date, the phlebotomist is required to check the armband and/or other qualifying documents, such as the requisition form, prior to drawing the patient's blood. Obtaining blood from the wrong patient constitutes an act of **negligence** (error or wrongdoing) and can result in disciplinary action.

Professionalism

Most people do not like having their blood drawn because of the potential discomfort, so **professionalism** and good interpersonal skills are critical attributes. Having a well-groomed and professional appearance demonstrates to others a sense of pride in oneself, the workplace, and one's overall profession.

TABLE 1-2 Two Common Collection Methods

Venipuncture	Insertion of needle into a vein to allow blood flow into a vacuum tube or syringe	
Dermal puncture	Use of a lancet or puncture device to prick the skin to remove small specimen of capillary blood	

Becoming certified or licensed as a phlebotomist can also send an important message to the patient and in turn the patient will have more confidence in your abilities. The patient will also perceive that you are an expert in your field. Membership in a professional organization will enhance the phlebotomist's professionalism by encouraging participation in continuing education activities such as workshops and seminars, and providing access to journals containing information regarding new developments in the field, as well as new regulations at the state and national levels.

Public Image

First impressions are very important. Your appearance is the first statement sent to those around you. Phlebotomists are expected to be clean, well groomed, and appropriately dressed for the work setting. Lack of good personal hygiene or proper dress can give a negative impression to an already anxious patient. Many institutions require that phlebotomists wear a lab jacket and specified shoes in order to meet **Occupational Safety and Health Administration (OSHA)** guidelines. OSHA is responsible for minimizing the risks and injuries to employees. Compliance with the dress code established by your facility is important for establishing a professional public image. Depending on the setting, the phlebotomist may be the only laboratory contact person a patient encounters, so a positive public image is important not only for the credibility of the individual, but for the laboratory department and institution as well.

Communication and Customer Service

The ability to communicate and provide customer service are important skills for the phlebotomist. Communication can be verbal or nonverbal. *Verbal* refs to the use of language or words to express ideas. The phlebotomist must be able to communicate using nonmedical terms so patients can understand what is being said to them. Some health professionals will continue to use medical terms in the presence of the patient. For example, using the term "venipuncture" with a patient instead of simply telling the patient that you will be "obtaining some blood" can create a block in communication. The phlebotomist must be capable of explaining procedures to patients of various ages in order to gain their confidence and cooperation. Never give false reassurance to patients by making statements such as, "You won't even feel it," because most patients feel some level of discomfort during phlebotomy procedures. Avoid using slang or "street" talk because different words have different meanings to different individuals. Address patients by name, avoiding inappropriate terms such as "honey" or "sweetie." Excessive talking is also to be avoided because it tends to be annoying to patients wanting and needing rest. It is best to speak using a calm and clear voice with a tone appropriate to patient need (e.g., a louder volume for a patient who is hard of hearing). The health care industry is service oriented, meaning that we want our customers (patients) to be pleased with both the services we provide and the manner in which they are delivered. This is customer service.

Patient Education & Communication

Using Proper Communication

The phlebotomist may be required to obtain blood from patients who are unable to communicate as a result of a stroke or other medical condition. Regardless of the patient's inability to communicate, the phlebotomist is expected to provide the same greetings, introductions, and explanations. The mere fact that a patient cannot respond does not necessarily mean that he or she cannot hear! Do not talk in the presence of comatose patients as if they cannot hear you.

Patients receive not only the spoken message but also the nonverbal cues sent by the phlebotomist (see Table 1-3). Nonverbal communication begins with attire and includes overall mannerisms or behaviors. Maintaining eye contact during patient interactions is a positive nonverbal response that assists with establishing trust. During the initial greeting, displaying a smile, maintaining erect body posture with relaxed arms, and avoiding the patient's personal space are usually well received. Personal space refers to the

TABLE 1-3 Nonverbal Communication: Positive versus Negative Gestures

Positive	Negative
• Good body posture • Eye contact • Neat, well-groomed appearance • Respecting personal space	• Drooping shoulders with head held low • Looking down or away from patient • Dingy, wrinkled lab coat; too much jewelry • Immediately approaching patient's space before greeting and explaining procedures

proximity or distance between individuals a person prefers when interacting with others. Many people feel uncomfortable when strangers approach them and enter their personal space. Appropriate distance for personal space or proximity varies based on gender, culture, and personal preference.

To provide positive communication and customer service, upon approaching any patient, the phlebotomist should properly introduce him- or herself, state the purpose of the visit, and request that the patient state his or her full name and date of birth. Patients will generally respond with a verbal or nonverbal gesture such as a nod of the head, indicating acknowledgment of the phlebotomist's presence. Once the initial greeting is established, it is acceptable and necessary to come in closer proximity to the patient's bedside or chair, depending on the workplace setting. In addition to professionalism and positive communication, customer service requires common courtesy. As mentioned earlier, when patients are having blood drawn, they may be anxious and not in the best of moods. They may be concerned about the results or just frightened. You can help their experience by being empathetic to their situation by observing their behavior, listening to their concerns, and addressing any situation promptly and effectively. You should approach any problem with flexibility and the obligation to find a resolution. For one example of proper customer service, see the Troubleshooting Box: Providing Customer Service.

Troubleshooting Providing Customer Service

The patients you draw blood from are your customers. Having patients is what provides you a job, so your patients/customers should be satisfied with your service. Customer service involves providing customer satisfaction through professionalism, positive communication, and an attitude that promotes resolution to problems when they occur.

Question: You are working alone in a busy laboratory because two other phlebotomists have called in sick. The laboratory waiting area is crowded. You expect another phlebotomist to arrive in about 20 minutes. What could you do to promote positive customer service?

_____

_____

_____

Checkpoint Questions 1-3

1. Name at least three duties and responsibilities of a phlebotomist.

_____

_____

_____

_____

2. A patient is having blood work done during her lunch hour and has waited 25 minutes before being called back for her blood to be drawn. How can you implement customer service in this situation?

_____

_____

_____

_____

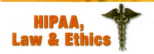 Answer the questions above and complete the *Roles and Responsibilities of the Phlebotomist* activity on the Student CD under Chapter 1 before you continue to the next section.

1-4 Where Do Phlebotomists Work?

There are two main categories of health care delivery systems in the United States, inpatient and outpatient services. Phlebotomists are employed in both of these settings as well as in select special settings. Hospitals, nursing homes, and rehabilitation centers are examples of inpatient facilities. Outpatient settings include physician offices, home health care agencies, ambulatory care centers, **reference laboratories** (off-site labs), and blood banks. Other special settings include veterinary offices, health maintenance organizations (HMOs), and the American Red Cross, to name a few.

HIPAA, Law & Ethics

Confidentiality

The phlebotomist may be privy to laboratory results. If you disclose results of any laboratory test, you will have breached patient confidentiality and may be subject to disciplinary or legal action or even a monetary fine.

Inpatient Facilities

Phlebotomists employed at inpatient facilities work directly with several members of the health care team (see Figure 1-4). Most hospitals have their own laboratories, which are referred to as "clinical" laboratories because they perform a wide range of tests in all specialties and subspecialties, such as

- **hematology** (the study of blood and blood-forming tissues)
- **microbiology** (the study of microscopic organisms)
- **chemistry** (the evaluation of the chemical constituents of the human body)
- **immunology** (the study of the body's resistance to disease and defense to foreign substances)
- **histology** (the study of human body tissues and cells)

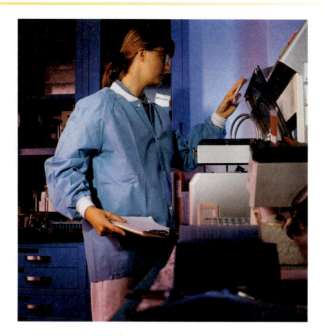

Figure 1-4 An inpatient laboratory is known as a clinical laboratory and performs a wide range of laboratory tests.

- **serology** (the identification of antibodies in the blood's serum)
- **urinalysis** (the examination of urine for physical, chemical, and microscopic characteristics)
- **toxicology** (the detection and study of the adverse effects of chemicals on living organisms)
- blood banking

Physicians order specific tests to assist with the evaluation of the patient's condition, and the phlebotomist's role is to collect the blood, properly label the specimen, and transport it to the laboratory. At some inpatient facilities, phlebotomists are also responsible for performing point-of-care testing, such as blood glucose monitoring. Point-of-care testing can assist the physician in making diagnoses more quickly, which often reduces the length of stay for hospitalized patients.

Being a member of the health care team may require that the phlebotomist assume other responsibilities such as basic patient care services at inpatient facilities. Some of these may include delivering meal trays and assisting with the transportation of patients from one department to another. Professional conduct must be exhibited at all times.

Outpatient Facilities

The fastest-growing outpatient settings are ambulatory care centers. These sites are walk-in facilities that patients can come to after business hours and on weekends. Lab tests are ordered to assist with the diagnosis and treatment of minor conditions. Outpatient laboratories usually perform tests involving chemistry, hematology, urinalysis, serology, and microbiology. Phlebotomists in these settings may also be responsible for performing other basic patient care duties such as obtaining vital signs and transporting patients for other procedures such as X rays.

Physician offices are also outpatient facilities. Phlebotomists or medical assistants certified in phlebotomy are usually responsible for collecting and

Figure 1-5 A physician office laboratory performs "waived" tests or ones that carry fewer risks to the patient.

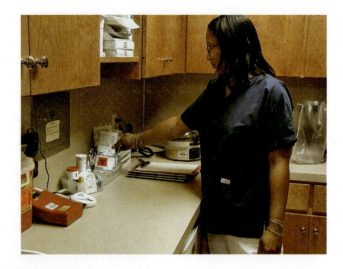

labeling a variety of specimens in the physician's office that are then transported to a reference laboratory for testing. In order for a physician's office laboratory to perform basic lab tests in their office, it must have "waived status" granted by the Clinical Laboratory Improvement Act (CLIA). A waived test is granted according to the difficulty in performing the test. Waived tests present much less risk to the patient because they performed on small amounts of blood or other specimens that are easier to obtain such as urine. The number of waived tests has increased. (See Figure 1-5.) Now tests such as nasal smears, for the presence of eosinophils to determine if infection is present, and cholesterol levels are approved in-office tests. So depending on the facility of employment, a phlebotomist may be required to perform some of these tests, as well as quality control checks on any test he or she performs.

Other outpatient facilities such as blood banks and the American Red Cross employ phlebotomists to collect blood. The blood collected will become a donor unit that might be used for a blood transfusion. Phlebotomists working for agencies are often hired to go into patient homes to collect blood specimens. As health care delivery systems continue to change, more care is being provided to patients in nursing homes and in their own residences. Some medical centers are now providing mobile venipuncture, where the phlebotomist goes to the patient's home to obtain blood specimens. Additionally, phlebotomists are hired by insurance agencies to perform in-home phlebotomy as a way of determining overall health before an insurance policy is written. Regardless of the work setting, proper collection, labeling, and handling of all specimens are critical to ensure accurate results and to prevent the need for having to repeat the test unnecessarily.

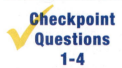

Checkpoint Questions 1-4

1. What is meant by a waived test and where would a waived test most likely be performed?

_____

_____

_____

_____

2. List and describe the common departments of a hospital laboratory.

_____

_____

_____

_____

_____

_____

Answer the questions above and complete the _Where Do Phlebotomists Work?_ activity on the Student CD under Chapter 1 before you continue to the next section.

1-5 Regulatory Agencies

Regulatory agencies routinely visit and inspect laboratories and medical offices to evaluate quality control and assurance. Laboratory facilities must have quality assurance programs in place to ensure that tests are effective and accurate. Quality assurance will be discussed in more detail in Chapter 7.

The 1988 **Clinical Laboratory Improvement Amendment (CLIA'88),** a revision of CLIA'67, was established to ensure that all laboratories receiving federal funds, regardless of size, type, or location, would meet the same standards and be certified by the federal government. This legislation, which became effective in 1992, serves as the main regulatory body for all laboratories, as well as establishing qualifications for phlebotomists. Classifications of laboratories are based on the complexity of testing performed and the associated patient risks if the tests are not performed properly. Some laboratories are categorized as "waived," and are not subject to inspections because they perform only simple tests that have minimal associated patient risks, such as dipstick urine testing. Other laboratories are classified as "moderately complex" or "highly complex," and both undergo inspections. Inspections are stricter for higher complexity laboratories. Personnel qualifications are specified for various levels of test complexity, which are outlined in the CLIA'88 regulations. Failure of any institution to comply with these regulations may result in termination of Medicare and Medicaid reimbursements, as well as loss of privilege to perform the procedure.

Hospital laboratories and physician office laboratories are governed by regulations that provide rules and guidelines for quality patient care. The Joint Commission on Accreditation of Healthcare Organizations (JCAHO) and the College of American Pathologists (CAP) are two accrediting agencies that help ensure a high standard of care for patients. The main accrediting agency for hospitals is the JCAHO. Physician offices must keep records for quality control, temperature readings, and equipment maintenance logs.

In addition to the federal government, other agencies responsible for overseeing aspects of the phlebotomy role include the **Centers for Disease Control and Prevention (CDC),** the Occupational Safety and Health Administration (OSHA), the Clinical and Laboratory Standards Institute

(CLSI), Healthcare Finance Administration (HCFA), and the Department of Health and Human Services (DHHS). Additional information about the role of regulatory agencies, certification, and accreditation is discussed in Chapter 7, Practicing Phlebotomy.

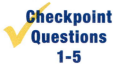

Checkpoint Questions 1-5

1. What was established to ensure the standards of laboratories?

   _____

   _____

   _____

2. What is the main accrediting agency for hospitals?

   _____

   _____

   _____

 Answer the questions above and complete the *Regulatory Agencies* activity on the Student CD under Chapter 1 before you continue to the next section.

1-6 Safety and Infection Control

Safety and infection control are two very important elements for protecting both you and the patient when you are providing any aspect of phlebotomy. The Centers for Disease Control and Prevention has set standards that prevent **nosocomial infections** (infections acquired in a hospital or other

Figure 1-6

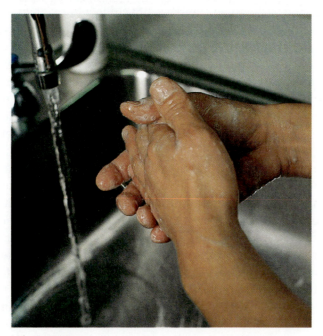

Handwashing.

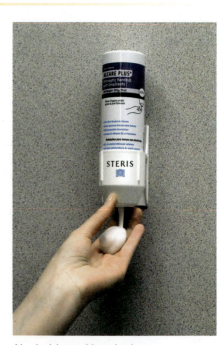

Alcohol-based hand rub.

medical setting). Nosocomial infections are responsible for about 20,000 deaths in the United States per year. Approximately 10% of American hospital patients (about two million every year) acquire a clinically significant nosocomial infection. Phlebotomists come in contact with many patients throughout the day, which makes performing correct hand hygiene critical (see Figure 1-6 and Table 1-4).

TABLE 1-4 Hand Hygiene Procedure Related to Phlebotomy

Recommended Practices

- Wash your hands with soap and water whenever they are visibly contaminated with blood or other body fluids.
- If hands are not visibly contaminated, an alcohol-based hand rub can be used.

Indications for Hand Hygiene

- Before and after putting on gloves
- Between patient contacts; between different procedures on same patient
- After touching blood, body fluids, secretions, excretions, and contaminated objects
- After handling specimen containers or tubes
- After restroom visits, eating, combing hair, handling money, and any other time your hands get contaminated

Basic Steps for Handwashing

- Remove all rings and jewelry.
- Turn on water and adjust temperature to warm.
- Wet hands liberally without leaning your body against sink area.
- Apply soap and work up a good lather.
- Use circular motions while applying friction, being sure to interlace fingers to clean between them for 2 minutes at the start of your work day, 10–15 seconds in between patients, and 1–2 minutes when hands are really soiled.
- Rinse each hand, allowing water to run from wrist toward fingertips, keeping fingers pointing downward. Contamination under fingernails should be removed with a tool designed for that purpose, such as an orange stick.
- Repeat above steps if hands are very soiled.
- Dry hands thoroughly with paper towels and discard them into waste receptacle.
- Turn off water with a clean, dry paper towel, if indicated.*
- Clean area using dry paper towels only if indicated.*

Basic Steps for Alcohol-Based Hand Cleanser

- Make sure there is no visible dirt or contamination.
- Apply ½ to 1 teaspoon of alcohol cleanser to one hand. Check the manufacturer's directions for proper amount.
- Rub your hands together vigorously, making sure all surfaces are covered.
- Continue rubbing until your hands are dry.

*Many facilities have sensors that turn water on automatically when the hands are lowered to the faucet. Other facilities have a knee or foot device that is used to turn the water on.

Figure 1-7 If one of the links in the chain of infection is broken, infection can be prevented.

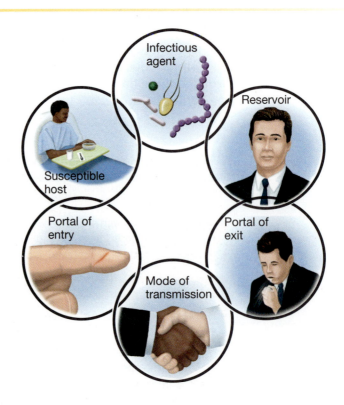

TABLE 1-5 Chain of Infection

Link	Description	How the Phlebotomist Can Break the Links
Infectious agent	Pathogen, or disease-producing microorganism	• Perform hand hygiene • Wear gloves when obtaining and handling any specimens • Dispose of contaminated materials properly • Use of personal protective equipment when required, including mask, gown, gloves, eye protection • Perform aseptic technique when required • Follow isolation precautions when required
Reservoir	Site where the organism grows and multiplies	
Portal of exit	The exit port for the pathogen to the host in the human includes skin, respiratory tract, and gastrointestinal tract	
Mode of transmission	How the pathogen travels; most commonly by contact, droplet, or airborne	
Portal of entry	Entry point for pathogen such as break in skin or respiratory system	
Susceptible host	Person at risk for developing an infection from the pathogen	

Nosocomial infections are prevented by hand hygiene and other precautions that break any of the links in the **chain of infection.** The chain of infection is six steps (links) that must take place for an infection to occur. The six links are the infectious agent, reservoir, portal of exit, mode of transmission, portal of entry, and susceptible host. Transmission of an infection can occur at any one of these six links in the chain of infection. Likewise, if the chain is broken at any of the links, an infection will not develop (see Figure 1-7 and Table 1-5).

Contact transmission is the most frequent source of nosocomial infections and can be by either direct or indirect contact. Direct contact requires a physical transfer of pathogens from reservoir to susceptible host (person to person) by something as simple as a touch.

Indirect contact occurs when a contaminated item, such as a soiled dressing, is handled prior to contact with a susceptible host (person to contaminated item to person). Indirect contact most often occurs when health care workers fail to wash their hands and change gloves between patients. Methicillin-resistant *Staphylococcus aureus* (MRSA) and *Clostridium difficile* (C-diff) enteritis are examples of infections spread by contact transmission.

Droplet transmission is a form of contact transmission, but the method of transfer is much different. This form occurs when droplets from an infected person are propelled short distances to the susceptible host through the nasal mucosa, mouth, or conjunctiva. Examples of infections spread by droplet transmission are influenza, mumps, and rubella. Droplets are propelled by coughing, sneezing, breathing, or talking. The droplets are not suspended in the air as they are with airborne transmission.

In airborne transmission, small particles carry the pathogens. These particles can be widely dispersed by air currents before being inhaled by a host. Legionnaires' disease, varicella, and tuberculosis are examples of infections spread by airborne transmission.

Vehicle-borne transmission occurs when a host comes in contact with a contaminated item such as food, linen, or equipment. To prevent this mode of transmission, soiled linen and equipment must be cleaned or disposed of properly. Vector-borne transmission requires an animal or insect as an agent to spread disease, such as the mosquito that carries the West Nile virus.

Preventing Infections

To help prevent nosocomial infections, the CDC in 1994 implemented two levels of precautions. The first level is **Standard Precautions** (formerly Universal Precautions). These precautions combine hand hygiene and the wearing of gloves when health care workers are exposed to blood and body fluids, nonintact skin, or mucous membranes. Standard Precautions include the major features of Universal Precautions, but they apply when workers are exposed to nonintact skin, mucous membranes, and blood and all body fluids, secretions, and excretions except sweat regardless of whether blood is visible. (Universal Precautions apply to blood and any other body fluids *only* if they contain visible blood.) The use of Standard Precautions reduces the risk of transmission of microorganisms from both recognized and unrecognized sources of infection. (See Appendix A: Standard Precautions.) In addition, the CDC advises that health care workers should not wear artificial nails because they are more likely to harbor gram-negative pathogens on their fingertips than workers with natural nails, both before and after handwashing. Natural nails should be no longer than one-fourth inch.

The CDC's second level of precautions is **isolation precautions** that are based on how the infectious agent is transmitted. These isolation precautions are

- Airborne precautions that require special air handling, ventilation, and additional respiratory protection (HEPA or N95 respirators)

- Droplet precautions that require mucous membrane protection (goggles and masks)
- Contact precautions that require gloves and gowns during direct skin-to-skin contact or contact with contaminated linen, equipment, and so on

You should follow Standard Precautions with every patient when performing phlebotomy. Isolation precautions are used less often and only with patients who have specific infections. When isolation precautions are mandated for a patient receiving phlebotomy, you will be required to follow the specific guidelines for the type of precautions implemented (see Appendix B: Transmission-Based Precautions).

The process of blood collection is an invasive procedure, and whenever blood or body fluid from one person comes in contact with another person, there is a major risk of exposure to bloodborne pathogens such as human immunodeficiency virus (HIV), hepatitis C virus (HCV), and hepatitis B virus (HBV). OSHA requires that health care facilities provide annual training on preventing exposure to bloodborne pathogens as well as the necessary **personal protective equipment (PPE)** for employee use, such as gloves, gowns, masks, and protective eyewear. (OSHA is the federal body charged with preventing or minimizing employee exposure to bloodborne pathogens, as outlined in the Occupational Exposure to Bloodborne Pathogens Standard.) See Figure 1-8 and Table 1-6 for more information about personal protective equipment and its applications.

In general when using PPE you should:

- Don before contact with the patient, generally before entering the room
- Use carefully—don't spread contamination
- Remove and discard carefully, either at the doorway or immediately outside patient room; remove respirator outside room
- Immediately perform hand hygiene

Figure 1-8 Removing gloves properly.

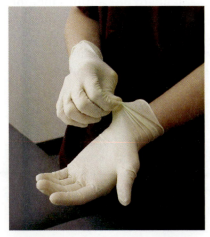 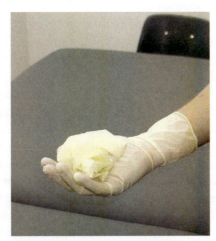 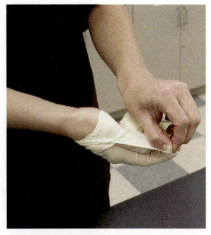

(a) Grasp the outside edge near the wrist. Peel away from the hand, turning the glove inside out. Hold the glove in opposite gloved hand.

(b) Hold the contaminated glove in the gloved hand while removing the second glove.

(c) Slide the ungloved finger under the wrist of the remaining glove. Peel off from inside, creating a bag for both gloves, and then discard.

TABLE 1-6 Personal Protective Equipment

Type	When Used	Rules for Use
Gloves	For hand contact with blood, mucous membranes, other potentially infectious materials, or when non-intact skin is anticipated, when performing vascular access procedures, or when handling contaminated items or surfaces	• Does not replace handwashing • Perform hand hygiene before applying and after removing gloves • When removing gloves do not touch the outside (contaminated) area of the gloves (see Figure 1-8) • Keep gloved hands away from the face • Avoid touching or adjusting other PPE • Remove if torn and perform hand hygiene before putting on new gloves • Limit surfaces and items touched • Extend gloves over isolation gown cuffs

Gown	During procedures and patient care activities when contact of clothing/exposed skin with blood/body fluids, secretions, or excretions is anticipated	• To put on gown
		  • Opening is in the back
		  • Secure at neck and waist
		• To remove gown
		  • Unfasten ties
		  • Peel gown away from neck and shoulder—do not touch outside
		  • Turn contaminated outside toward the inside
		  • Fold or roll into a bundle
		  • Discard

Mask	During patient care activities likely to generate splashes or sprays of blood, body fluids, secretions, or excretions	• Must fully cover nose and mouth
		• Respirator masks such as N95, N99, and N100 must be used for airborne precautions
		• To put on mask
		  • Place over nose, mouth, and chin
		  • Fit flexible nosepiece over nose bridge
		  • Secure on head with ties or elastic
		  • Adjust to fit
		• To remove mask
		  • Untie the bottom, then top tie
		  • Remove from face—do not touch the outside
		  • Discard

Eye protection	During patient care activities likely to generate splashes or sprays of blood, body fluids, secretions, or excretions	• Goggles should fit snugly over and around the eyes
		• Personal glasses are not an acceptable substitute
		• Can use a face shield that protects face, nose, mouth, and eyes
		• Face shield should cover forehead, extend below chin, and wrap around side of face
		• Position goggles over eyes and secure to the head using the earpieces or headband
		• Position face shield over face and secure on brow with headband
		• Remove goggles or face shield
		  • Grasp ear or head pieces with ungloved hands
		  • Lift away from face—do not touch outside
		  • Place in designated receptacle for reprocessing or disposal

- Apply in correct sequence; gown, mask or respirator, goggles or face shield, then gloves
- Remove in correct sequence; gloves, face shield or goggles, gown, then mask or respirator

Employees at increased risk of exposure are to receive, free of charge, the HBV (hepatitis B virus) vaccination. Each health care facility is also required to have an occupational exposure plan, which is a protocol to be followed in the event an employee is exposed to bloodborne pathogens. The ultimate objective is to protect patients, peers, and oneself from coming in contact with potentially harmful materials such as contaminated needles and syringes. Proper disposal of venipuncture equipment greatly decreases the incidence of accidental needlestick injuries and exposure.

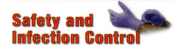

Safety and Infection Control

Isolation Precaution Equipment

Follow the guidelines for isolation precautions when entering a patient's room. If you are not certain what personal protective equipment (PPE) to wear, such as gowns, gloves, or mask, consult with the licensed practitioner caring for the patient, such as a nurse. *Never* take a tray of phlebotomy equipment into an isolation room. Take only the equipment needed for the particular draw. If you need additional equipment, you must remove all PPE before leaving the room, collect the needed supplies, then don new PPE before re-entering the room. Only the equipment to be used should be taken in, and only the tubes and the phlebotomist should leave the room. Any unused equipment or supplies must be left in the room.

Needlestick Injuries

The National Institute for Occupational Safety and Health (NIOSH) estimates that between 600,000 and 800,000 needlestick injuries occur annually, exposing health care workers to bloodborne pathogens. A needlestick has both financial and emotional consequences. Follow-up for a high-risk exposure is approximately $500 to $1000 per needlestick even if no infection develops. However, the emotional impact and health consequences can be severe and can continue for a long time, especially if the exposure is to HIV. Needlestick injuries are preventable with proper education, safer equipment, and elimination of the need for needles whenever possible.

Through the recommendation of NIOSH and the efforts of OSHA, the Needlestick Safety and Prevention Act was passed into law in 2001. The intent of the law and the implementation regulation is to mandate the use of safety devices that reduce needlestick injuries in the clinical setting. The introduction of needleless equipment and protected needles has significantly reduced the risk of needlestick injuries. All devices selected for phlebotomy should be equipped with needlestick prevention features. These devices will be discussed in more detail in Chapter 3, Equipment for Specimen Collection.

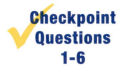

1. Name three things you can do to prevent infection.

_____

_____

_____

_____

2. In what order should you apply and remove PPE?

_____

_____

_____

_____

Answer the questions above and complete the *Safety and Infection Control* activity on the Student CD under Chapter 1 before you continue to the next section.

1-7 HIPAA, Ethics, and Law

In 1996, the **Health Insurance Portability and Accountability Act (HIPAA)** was established in response to information that was being transferred electronically for medical transactions. In 2003, a federal law was passed that establishes a national standard for electronic health care transactions and protects the privacy and **confidentiality** of patient information. Among other provisions, HIPAA states that information about a patient must not be discussed with individuals other than the patient unless the patient has given written or verbal permission for you to do so. A patient's information cannot be shared among health care professionals unless it is for the patient's treatment. The following is a list of other guidelines from HIPAA that could apply to the care of patients during phlebotomy.

- Close patients' room doors when caring for them or discussing their health.
- Do not talk about patients in public places.
- Turn computer screens that contain patient information so passersby cannot see the information.
- Log off computers when you are done.
- Do not walk away from patient medical records; close them when leaving.

Following a code of ethics is a principal part of being a phlebotomist. **Ethics** consists of a set of written rules, procedures, or guidelines that examines values, actions, and choices to help determine right from wrong. It is also a moral philosophy that varies by individual, religion, social status, or heritage. Acting morally toward others requires putting yourself in their place. If you were a patient requiring blood tests to rule out a disease or other condition, how would you want to be treated?

There may be instances when the patient or family member will ask the phlebotomist why the blood is being drawn, or what the results of previous blood tests were. It is the responsibility of the physician to discuss this information with the patient, not that of the phlebotomist. In such cases, the phlebotomist might respond by saying, "You will need to ask your physician about these tests or results. I am not allowed to discuss them with you." All information concerning the care of patients is strictly confidential and is not to be discussed. Inpatient settings may require the phlebotomist to travel throughout the facility to collect specimens, from the patient's bedside to other departments such as the emergency room. Information obtained, no matter how small, must remain confidential to protect the patient and the facility.

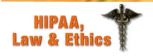

Obtaining a Blood Specimen

With few exceptions, phlebotomists will be required to obtain blood specimens when ordered by the primary practitioner regardless of the patient diagnosis. Patients with infectious diseases such as tuberculosis, hepatitis, and AIDS deserve to have their blood drawn just as other patients would. Some health care personnel attempt to avoid such patients. This is considered discrimination and may result in disciplinary actions and/or legal liability. All patients, regardless of condition, should be treated with respect and dignity. Certain exceptions could occur when a phlebotomist may not be required to draw a specimen, such as when a patient is receiving radiation treatment and the phlebotomist is pregnant, or when an irate patient infected with hepatitis or AIDS does not have the phlebotomist's safety at hand.

Consent is an important legal aspect of phlebotomy. Prior to performing any blood collection procedure, the phlebotomist must explain to the patient in nonmedical terms what he or she can expect to happen during the procedure. Patients generally sign a consent form for treatment during the initial in-take before entering the hospital or before being treated by a physician in his or her office. Consents take a variety of forms, for example, written agreements, spoken words, implicit actions, or making an appointment for a test. It is important to provide quality patient education and to make sure the patient understands what he or she is agreeing to. Because the phlebotomist will also be instrumental in collecting urine specimens for chain of custody, it is essential to discuss expressed consent whereby the patient not only has to be informed of the procedure and its process, but he or she must also sign a consent form agreeing to have the procedure done. Other procedures that may require written consent would be drug and alcohol screens and HIV testing.

The issue of patient rights is not new, and it has been clearly defined since 1975 by the American Hospital Association in a document called the **Patient's Bill of Rights.** In addition to the right to refuse care, patients have the right to be treated with respect, to have all records and information classified as confidential, to be informed about the purpose and expected results of treatments, and to have access to their medical records.

On occasion, family members can serve to calm the patient prior to procedures, but there are times when the visitors may interfere with the blood collection process. If there are too many visitors or if they appear to make the patient anxious, politely request that they leave the room for a few minutes. It is rare that visitors will resent such a request when asked politely.

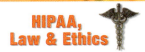

Consent

Consent must always be very clear. If a patient just puts out his or her arm, but does not bother to stop watching TV or otherwise acknowledge the phlebotomist, this is considered implied consent. If the patient doesn't speak English, but notices the tray and automatically puts his or her arm out, that too is considered implied consent. Only if conflicting information is present, or if the patient doesn't understand English and seems confused about what you are there for, must the phlebotomist be very careful to verify the true intent of the patient. Conflicting consent has resulted in several lawsuits. If a minor child or mentally incompetent patient is to have blood drawn, and the parent or guardian is not present, the written consent for treatment the parent signed on admission is considered adequate. There are three instances where a patient can **NOT** refuse to consent. These are in the case of a minor or a patient under the age of 18, a patient with mental incapacitation, or a patient who has been ordered by law to have his or her blood drawn.

Phlebotomists may also be confronted with issues involving team members. Serving as a member of a team is a challenge because all the "players" affect the outcome. The team concept implies working together to achieve common goals. Phlebotomists will work closely with other phlebotomists, physicians, nurses, and other health care members. The ultimate goal is to provide quality care to consumers accessing your health care facility.

All blood specimen tubes must be properly labeled at the patient's bedside. If you find specimen tubes without a label, bring this to the attention of other team members. Do not label specimens that you did not collect. If you label a specimen as requested by a team member, you become accountable for the accuracy of that specimen. Unless you saw your team member obtain the specimen, you cannot be sure that the blood specimen belongs to that patient. Just imagine the potential implications of placing the wrong patient label on a specimen. A patient with a potential abnormal test result may not receive the needed treatment, and a patient not needing that treatment may receive it. Both of these situations could lead to disciplinary actions and compromise patient safety, so never label specimens for which you did not assume responsibility.

Patient Refusal

The phlebotomist may encounter a patient who refuses to have blood drawn. In such instances, it is best to remind the patient that the physician ordered the tests to assist with evaluating the patient's condition. If this explanation fails and the patient still refuses to have his or her blood drawn, politely leave the room and be sure to document a detailed account of the patient interaction. It is also helpful in hospital settings to tell the patient's nurse so the physician can be notified as soon as possible.

As a phlebotomist it is important to protect yourself against harm from blood and body fluid exposure as well as legal issues. If you feel as though there are policies and procedures that will place your safety in jeopardy, you must first alert your supervisor. If there is no resolution, take it to the next person in charge until your situation has been resolved. Phlebotomists may also purchase liability insurance through several insurance carriers who provide low-cost coverage to health care workers. Be sure to check with your employer to see if they carry liability coverage on you; if so, then there would be no need to purchase liability insurance.

Checkpoint Questions 1-7

1. Name three ways you can follow HIPAA guidelines as a phlebotomist.

   _____

   _____

   _____

   _____

2. What should you say to a patient who asks you for the results of a blood test?

   _____

   _____

   _____

   _____

Answer the questions above and complete the *HIPAA, Ethics, and Law* activity on the Student CD under Chapter 1 before you continue to the next section.

Chapter Summary

- Phlebotomy has evolved from the use of leeches for blood collection to modern-day certified phlebotomists.
- Phlebotomists are responsible for the collection, processing, and transportation of blood specimens.
- Professionalism includes such things as a positive attitude and appearance plus keeping up with current information in the field. Public image starts with the first impression and is expressed in your behavior and methods of communication. Communication and customer service are necessary to maintain your public image and confidence and cooperation from your supervisor, patients, and co-workers.
- Phlebotomists can be employed at hospitals, rehabilitation centers, nursing homes, clinics, physicians' offices, ambulatory care centers, blood banks, and reference laboratories.
- The regulating agencies for phlebotomy include CLSI, JCAHO, HCFA, DHHS, CDC, and OSHA.
- Infection control and safety practices include hand hygiene, gloving, Standard Precautions, and isolation precautions.
- HIPAA provides protection of health care information. Ethics consists of a set of rules, procedures, or guidelines that helps determine right from wrong. The law includes following your scope of practice, policies, and procedures at your facility and obtaining consent for phlebotomy procedures.

Chapter Review

Multiple Choice

Choose the best answer for each question.

1. The term *phlebotomy* comes from Greek words that translate to mean:
   a. Draw blood
   b. Cut a vein
   c. Drain blood
   d. Dermal cut

2. Phlebotomy may be used to help treat which of the following medical conditions?
   a. Polycythemia
   b. Diabetes
   c. Hypertension
   d. Anemia

3. The main duty of a phlebotomist is to:
   a. Interpret laboratory values
   b. Evaluate blood specimens
   c. Process blood specimens
   d. Collect blood specimens

4. If a phlebotomist failed to properly identify a patient and blood was drawn on the wrong patient, this would be considered an act of:
   a. Malpractice
   b. Assault and battery
   c. Negligence
   d. Consent

5. CLIA classifies laboratories based on:
   a. Number of employees
   b. Size of the laboratory
   c. Number of tests performed
   d. Complexity of tests performed

6. Which of the following is the current CDC guideline for infection control?
   a. Universal Precautions
   b. Standard Precautions
   c. Body Substance Isolation
   d. Waived Precautions

7. A phlebotomist must obtain _____ before he or she draws a patient's blood.
   a. a license
   b. hepatitis B vaccination
   c. certification
   d. consent

8. If your hands are visibly soiled, you can:
   a. Use an alcohol-based hand rub
   b. Perform handwashing
   c. Wear gloves
   d. Perform phlebotomy

9. Customer service would least likely include the following:
   a. Flexibility
   b. Professionalism
   c. Common courtesy
   d. Complexity

10. Which of the following is the most frequent source of nosocomial infections?
    a. Direct or indirect contact
    b. HIV
    c. Airborne particles
    d. Droplet particles

Fill in the Blanks

Write the word(s) or statement needed to answer the following questions.

11. List two negative verbal and nonverbal communication skills that must be avoided.

   Verbal   *Nonverbal*

   _____   _____

   _____   _____

12. List three settings in which a phlebotomist may gain employment.

   _____

   _____

   _____

13. What term describes tests that are performed at the patient's bedside?

   _____

   _____

True or False

Write T or F on the line provided to indicate whether you think each statement is true or false. Correct the false statements to make them true.

_____ 14. Entry into phlebotomy programs usually requires a high school diploma or its equivalent.

   _____

_____ **15.** Phlebotomists are the only health care personnel allowed to collect blood specimens.

_____ **16.** Venipuncture requires the use of a skin puncture device to remove a small amount of capillary blood.

_____ **17.** Blood specimens assist in the diagnosing and monitoring of patients.

_____ **18.** All specimens require proper collection, handling, labeling, and transporting.

_____ **19.** A HEPA mask is used for airborne precautions.

_____ **20.** Dermal puncture is used for larger blood samples.

Matching

Match each agency, legislature, or committee abbreviation with the correct description by writing the appropriate letter in the space provided.

_____ **21.** JCAHO

_____ **22.** CLIA

_____ **23.** CDC

_____ **24.** CLSI

_____ **25.** OSHA

a. Federal agency responsible for monitoring and reporting diseases.

b. Nonprofit organization that sets standards for phlebotomy training programs.

c. Federal body responsible for preventing or minimizing work-related injuries.

d. Main accrediting agency for hospitals.

e. Legislation responsible for regulating all laboratories and phlebotomists.

What Should You Do? _Critical Thinking Application_

Use your critical thinking skills to respond to the following situations.

26. A phlebotomist has been asked to obtain a blood specimen from a hospitalized patient. The phlebotomist enters the patient's room and gives the appropriate greeting, only to discover that the patient speaks only Spanish, a language the phlebotomist is unfamiliar with. Should the phlebotomist proceed with the blood collection? What are the phlebotomist's next steps? Give information to support your answer such as legal/ethical implications and also consider the patient's rights.

_____

_____

_____

_____

27. While explaining the purpose of a visit to a patient, the phlebotomist notices five visitors entering the room. The patient greets the visitors pleasantly, and one of the visitors asks the phlebotomist what blood tests have been ordered. How should the phlebotomist handle this situation and why?

_____

_____

_____

_____

28. The phlebotomist is scheduled to obtain a blood specimen from a patient in a patient's home. The phlebotomist enters the home and makes the appropriate greetings. The patient is very agitated and states, "I'm just sick and tired of you people drawing my blood. It's not helping me to get any better, so get out! I refuse to be a pincushion for you medical jerks!" What would be a good response for the phlebotomist to make? How should the phlebotomist handle this situation?

_____

_____

_____

_____

29. A phlebotomist employed at the outpatient clinic of a large acute-care hospital begins her shift to find the waiting room full of patients. Two of the scheduled phlebotomists have called in sick, and it will be at least 20 minutes before any additional phlebotomists can arrive. The phlebotomist begins to call patients back and listens while each patient voices his or her frustration, saying only what is required to collect the specimen and letting the patients leave. Did the phlebotomist make any error? What could he or she have done differently?

_____

_____

_____

_____

30. You notice a co-worker carrying a tray of phlebotomy equipment out of the room of a patient who is in airborne precautions. What should you do?

_____

_____

_____

_____

Get Connected *Internet Activity*

Visit the McGraw-Hill Higher Education Online Learning Center *Phlebotomy for Healthcare Personnel* Website at **www.mhhe.com/healthcareskills** to complete the following activities.

The History of Bloodletting To find out more about the history of bloodletting and the equipment used, search the Internet and find at least one image to share with the class:

- UCLA Biomedical Library has graphics of bloodletting devices and historical data
- Museum of Questionable Medical Devices by Graham Ford presents an overview of ancient bloodletting practices

Phlebotomy Regulating Agencies To find out more about phlebotomy, visit any of these sites:
- American Society for Clinical Pathology
- American Society of Phlebotomy Technicians
- National Credentialing Agency
- National Phlebotomy Association
- American Medical Technologis
- Centers for Disease Control and Prevention
- Occupational Safety and Health Administration
- Joint Commission on Accreditation of Healthcare Organizations
- College of American Pathologists
- National Healthcareer Association
- National Center for Competency Testing

Research one site and determine its mission and relationship to the practice of phlebotomy. Share your findings with your class.

 ## Using the Student CD

Now that you have completed the material in the chapter text, return to the Student CD and complete any chapter activities you have not yet done. Practice your terminology with the "Key Term Concentration" game. Review the chapter material with the "Spin the Wheel" game. Take the final chapter test and complete the troubleshooting question. E-mail or print your results to document your proficiency for this chapter.

2 Blood Circulation, Function, and Composition

Learning Outcomes

Upon completion of this chapter, you should be able to:

- Describe circulation and the purpose of the vascular system.
- Discuss three types of circulation.
- List and describe the three layers of blood vessels.
- Identify and describe the structures and functions of the different types of blood vessels.
- Locate and name the veins most commonly used for phlebotomy procedures.
- List the functions of blood.
- Identify the major components of blood.
- Describe the major function of red blood cells, white blood cells, and platelets.
- List the different types of white blood cells and give the function of each.
- Differentiate between serum and plasma.
- Define hemostasis and describe the basic coagulation process.
- Describe how ABO and Rh blood types are determined.

Key Terms

agglutination	atrium (atria, pl.)
antecubital fossa	basilic vein
antibody	basophil
anticoagulant	blood type
antigen	capillary
aorta	centrifugation
arteriole	cephalic vein
artery	coagulation

cytoplasm	phagocytosis
deoxygenated	plasma
diapedesis	pulmonary artery
eosinophil	pus
erythrocyte	Rh antigen
fibrin	septum
fibrinogen	serum
hematoma	thrombin
hemoglobin	thrombocyte
hemostasis	tunica adventitia
leukocyte	tunica intima
lymphocyte	tunica media
median cubital vein	vein
monocyte	vena cava
neutrophil	ventricles
oxygenated	venule

2-1 Introduction

The average adult body contains about 8 to 12 pints of blood. Blood is distributed through more than 70,000 miles of tubes known as the vascular system. If these tubes were lined up end to end, they would reach between New York City and San Francisco over 24 times. Blood is the transporting fluid for the body. Blood's composition is complex and essential to sustaining life.

The phlebotomist must have an understanding of the circulation of blood and its composition and functions. In addition to the cellular and liquid composition of blood, the phlebotomist must know how the closed circuit of blood vessels transports blood. Knowing the location of blood vessels, especially the most commonly used arm veins, and the composition of blood is essential to performing venipuncture.

Checkpoint Question 2-1

1. Name at least three things the phlebotomist should know about blood function and composition.

_____

_____

_____

_____

2-2 Circulation and the Vascular System

The human vascular system consists of several tubelike structures called blood vessels. These tubes, which vary in size and structure, are all interconnected, forming a closed circuit. This closed circuit, along with the heart, is responsible for the circulation of blood.

The heart is a large muscle responsible for pumping the blood through the vascular system. If you look inside the heart, you see a wall of muscle that

Figure 2-1 The heart is a muscular pump with four chambers that distributes the blood to the lungs and the body.

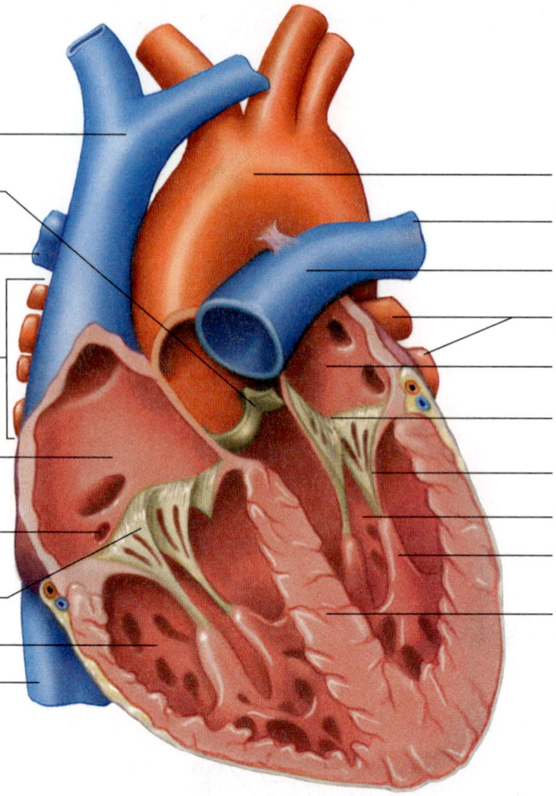

divides it down the middle, into a left half and a right half. This muscular wall is called a **septum.** Another wall separates the rounded top part of the heart from the cone-shaped bottom part. So there are actually four chambers (spaces) inside the heart. Each top chamber is called an **atrium** (plural: atria). The bottom chambers are called **ventricles.** The atria are often referred to as holding chambers, while the ventricles are called pumping chambers (see Figure 2-1).

Blood can flow from the atria down into the ventricles because there are openings in the walls that separate them. These openings are called *valves* because they open in one direction like trapdoors to let the blood pass through. Then they close, so the blood cannot flow backward into the atria. With this system, blood always flows in only one direction inside the heart. There are also valves at the bottom of the large arteries that carry blood away from the heart: the **aorta** and the **pulmonary artery.** These valves keep the blood from flowing backward into the heart once it has been pumped out.

The heart and vascular system are responsible for transportation of blood through the heart, lungs, and body. These three types of circulation are known as coronary (heart), pulmonary (lungs), and systemic (body) (see Figure 2-2).

Coronary Circulation

Coronary circulation provides the blood supply to the heart. Oxygenated blood travels from the left ventricle through the aorta directly into the coronary arteries. There are two main coronary arteries (left and right). The left main artery has more branches because the left side of the heart is more muscular and requires more blood supply. The deoxygenated blood travels through the coronary veins and is collected in the coronary sinus, which empties the blood directly into the right atrium.

Figure 2-2   The right side of the heart pumps blood to the lungs (pulmonary circulation). The left side of the heart delivers blood to the body (systemic circulation).

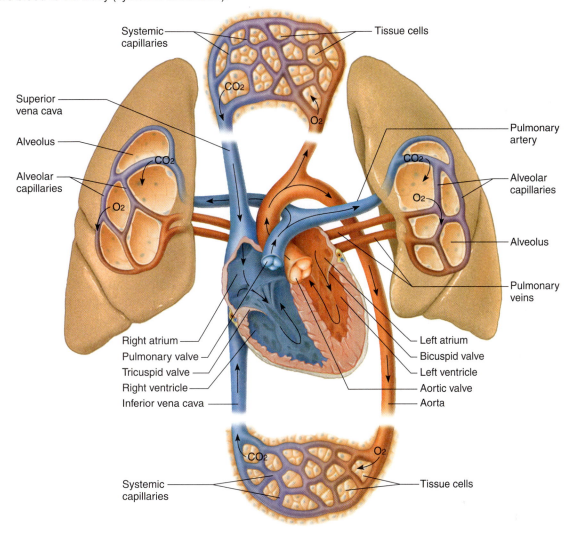

Pulmonary Circulation

Pulmonary circulation occurs when blood that has been used by the body's cells is returned back to the heart and transported to the lungs. The lung vascular network is where this **deoxygenated** blood (having a higher concentration of carbon dioxide than oxygen) becomes **oxygenated** (having more oxygen than carbon dioxide). The pulmonary arteries deliver the deoxygenated blood to the lungs. This blood is cleansed through the process of respiration within the lungs. Pulmonary circulation is also charged with returning this oxygenated blood back to the heart, so that it can be pumped throughout the body. The blood returns to the heart through the pulmonary veins.

Systemic Circulation

The systemic circulation of the vascular system is responsible for delivering nutrient-rich, oxygenated blood to all other parts of the body. The network of blood vessels picks up essential nutrients from the digestive tract to feed body cells. After delivering nutrients and oxygenated blood, systemic circulation removes waste products from body cells and tissues before transporting this blood back to the heart. Blood returning to the heart from the body thus contains waste products, such as carbon dioxide, that must be cleansed by the lungs. Blood containing a greater amount of carbon dioxide than oxygen is referred to as venous blood. Venous blood is pumped by the heart to the lungs, where oxygen is absorbed into the blood and a large amount of carbon dioxide is removed from the blood. Once the exchange of gases (oxygen and carbon dioxide) has taken place, this blood becomes known as arterial blood. All blood, both venous and arterial, is transported through the circular network of the vascular system by blood vessels through the heart and lungs.

Blood flows from the body to the superior and inferior vena cava, then empties into the right atrium. Blood then flows through the tricuspid valve into the right ventricle. Blood leaves the right ventricle and goes through the pulmonary semilunar valve, and the pulmonary arteries pick it up and take it to the lungs. From the lungs it travels by way of pulmonary veins and empties into the left atrium. Blood then flows through the mitral or bicuspid valve into the left ventricle. Blood leaves the left ventricle and goes through the aortic semilunar valve to the aorta into the coronary circulation and to the rest of the body.

Circulation of Blood

Oxygenated blood is transported from the heart by the largest **artery,** the aorta, which branches into smaller arteries, which further branch to become even smaller in size (**arterioles**), until they reach the **capillaries,** the smallest of all the blood vessels. Here in the capillaries, gas exchange takes place. Oxygenated blood enters the tissues by way of these small capillaries. In addition to delivering oxygenated blood and nutrients, the capillaries absorb waste products. These microscopic vessels, carrying deoxygenated blood, then connect to the smallest of the veins (**venules**), which continue to enlarge into larger vessels (**veins**), until the largest of all veins, the superior and inferior **vena cava,** returns this blood to the heart. This cycle continues over and over again, with blood traveling through each of the body's blood vessels forming a circular vascular network (see Figure 2-3).

Checkpoint Question 2-2

1. Name and briefly describe three types of circulation.

_____

_____

_____

_____

_____

 Answer the question above and complete the *Circulation and the Vascular Systems* activity on the Student CD under Chapter 2 before you continue to the next section.

Figure 2-3 Arteries carry oxygen-rich blood through capillaries where gas exchange occurs. Veins carry deoxygenated blood back to the heart.

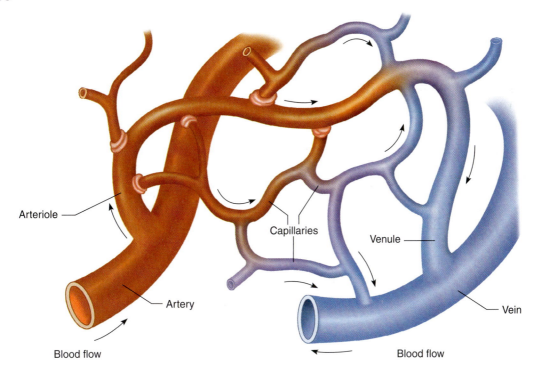

Arteriole

Capillaries

Venule

Artery

Vein

Blood flow

Blood flow

2-3 Blood Vessels

There are three main types of blood vessels: arteries, veins, and capillaries. Arteries are vessels that transport blood away from the heart, and veins carry blood toward the heart. In the human body, all arteries *except* the pulmonary arteries contain oxygenated blood, and all veins *except* the pulmonary veins carry deoxygenated blood. The pulmonary arteries transport deoxygenated blood away from the heart to the lungs. The pulmonary veins carry oxygenated blood from the lungs back to the heart. The important fact to remember is that all arteries carry blood away from the heart, and all veins transport blood toward the heart. Arteries branch into smaller arteries called arterioles, and veins branch into smaller veins known as venules. The third major classification of blood vessels, capillaries, are the smallest and most numerous blood vessels in the human body. Capillaries serve as a connecting point between the smallest arteries (arterioles) and smallest veins (venules). Capillaries are unique in that they are only one cell layer thick, which permits the exchange of oxygen and carbon dioxide. These thin-walled, tiny vessels are the only sites for gas exchange to take place in the body.

Structure of Blood Vessels

Blood vessels are structured to perform specific functions. Arteries and veins are composed of three layers of tissue (see Figure 2-4):

- **Tunica intima**—the innermost, smooth layer in direct contact with the blood
- **Tunica media**—the middle, thickest layer, capable of contracting and relaxing

Figure 2-4 Arteries and veins are composed of three layers of tissue.

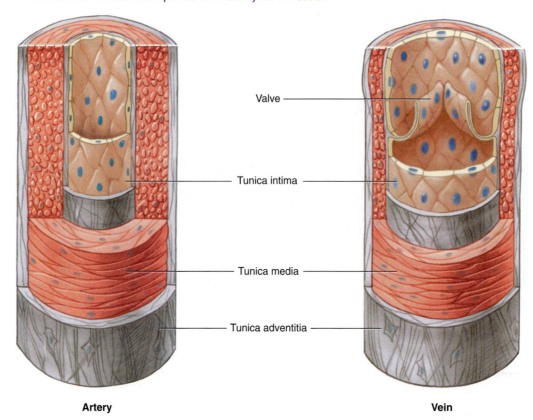

Valve

Tunica intima

Tunica media

Tunica adventitia

Artery   **Vein**

- **Tunica adventitia**—the outer covering, which serves to protect and support the vessel

Capillaries, the third type of blood vessel, are comprised of only one layer of tissue. This single-layer vessel is so small that blood cells have to pass through it in single file. The reason for such thin, small vessels is to facilitate the exchange of gases and nutrients. Water and other dissolved substances can be exchanged in the tissues as a result of the capillary structure.

Arteries

Arteries always carry blood away from the heart (efferent). Arteries carry oxygenated blood, with the exception of the pulmonary artery. Arteries transport blood under high pressure. They are elastic, muscular, and thick walled. Artery walls are much thicker than the walls of your capillaries and veins. Many arteries in the body are paired, meaning that there is a left and right artery with the same name (see Figure 2-5).

The alternating expansion and narrowing of the arterial walls, caused by the contraction and relaxation of the heart, creates what we refer to as a pulse, which can be felt at specific sites on the body. Arterial blood is bright red due to the high level of oxygen, and it flows with a much greater pressure or force than does venous blood. This increase in pressure is produced by the heart, as blood is being pumped out of the heart, through the arteries,

Figure 2-5 Arteries carry blood away from the heart.

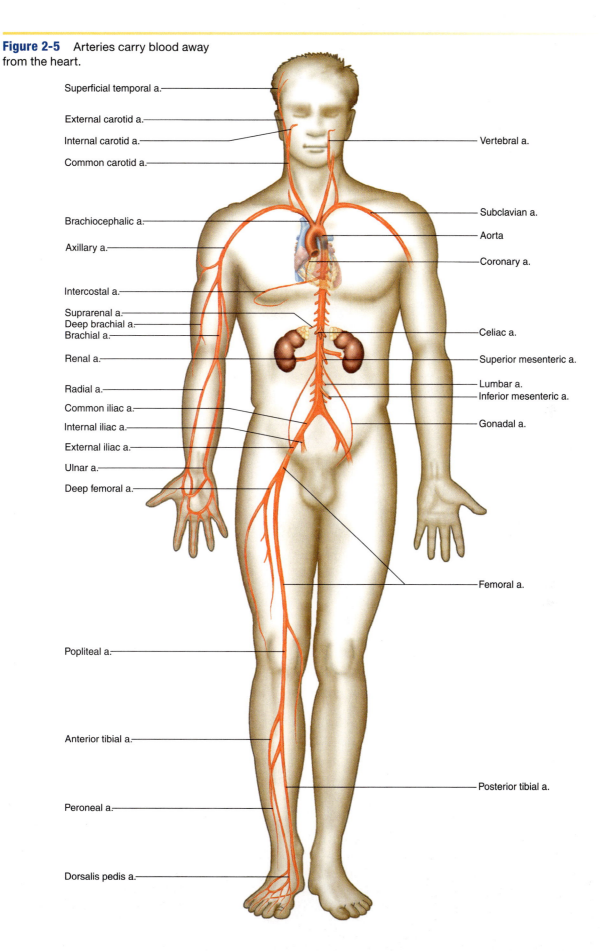

Superficial temporal a.

External carotid a.

Internal carotid a.

Common carotid a.

Vertebral a.

Brachiocephalic a.

Axillary a.

Subclavian a.

Aorta

Coronary a.

Intercostal a.

Suprarenal a.
Deep brachial a.
Brachial a.

Celiac a.

Renal a.

Superior mesenteric a.

Radial a.

Lumbar a.
Inferior mesenteric a.

Common iliac a.

Internal iliac a.

Gonadal a.

External iliac a.

Ulnar a.

Deep femoral a.

Femoral a.

Popliteal a.

Anterior tibial a.

Posterior tibial a.

Peroneal a.

Dorsalis pedis a.

Figure 2-6 Veins carry blood toward the heart.

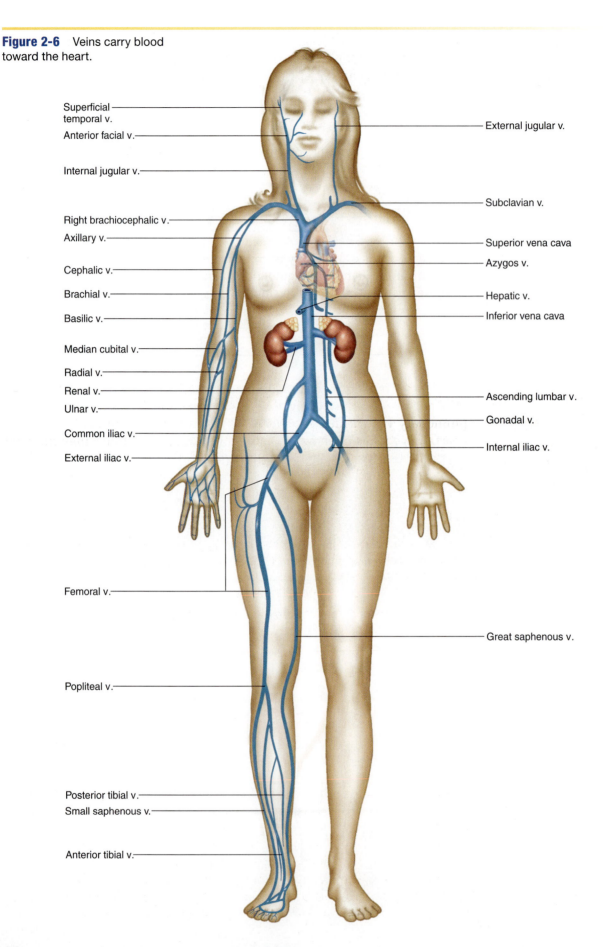

Superficial temporal v.

Anterior facial v.

Internal jugular v.

Right brachiocephalic v.

Axillary v.

Cephalic v.

Brachial v.

Basilic v.

Median cubital v.

Radial v.

Renal v.

Ulnar v.

Common iliac v.

External iliac v.

Femoral v.

Popliteal v.

Posterior tibial v.

Small saphenous v.

Anterior tibial v.

External jugular v.

Subclavian v.

Superior vena cava

Azygos v.

Hepatic v.

Inferior vena cava

Ascending lumbar v.

Gonadal v.

Internal iliac v.

Great saphenous v.

and to the body. The thickness of arterial walls allows for the transport of blood under such high pressure. Arteries branch into smaller vessels, arterioles, then into capillaries.

Capillaries

Capillaries are the smallest blood vessels and provide a link from arterioles to venules. All gas exchange occurs at this level. Capillaries can only be seen through a microscope. Capillary walls are extremely thin to allow for selective permeability of various cells and substances. Nutrients, molecules, and oxygen pass out of the capillaries and into surrounding cells and tissues. Waste products like carbon dioxide and nitrogenous waste pass from the cells and tissues of the body back into the bloodstream for excretion from the respiratory, urinary, integumentary, and digestive systems. (For a review of these systems and other systems of the body, see Appendix C, Review of Body Systems.)

Veins

Veins are blood vessels that carry deoxygenated blood toward the heart (afferent vessels). (See Figure 2-6.) There is one exception, and that is the pulmonary vein, which transports oxygenated blood from the lungs to the heart. Large veins often have the same names as the arteries they run next to. However there are exceptions to the rule. Veins flow against gravity in many areas of the body. They have one-way valves and use weak muscular action to move the blood cells. Figure 2-7 shows a one-way valve flow. The pressure from the heart is diminished by the time the blood reaches the veins so the pressure is not as forceful as it is in the arteries.

Another important function of veins is to serve as a reservoir. About 65% to 70% of the body's total blood volume is stored in the veins. This blood is darker in color and flows in a slow, oozing manner, unlike the fast, pulsating flow of arterial blood. Because veins store a large amount of blood, have thinner walls, and have low pressure, veins are the vessels of choice for the collection of blood.

Toward heart

(a)   (b)

Figure 2-7 One-way valves, found only in veins, permit blood to flow back toward the heart.

Troubleshooting

Artery or Vein?

It is important to know how to tell the difference between an artery and a vein, and what happens when you puncture an artery. When finding a venipuncture site, remember that a vein will feel bouncy or have a resiliency to it, and an artery will feel firmer and actually pulsate. In the event of an accidental puncturing of an artery, the blood will appear bright red instead of dark red, and the flow is usually more forceful. If this occurs, immediately withdraw the needle and apply firm pressure for at least five minutes, then apply a taut gauze dressing. Instruct the patient to keep the arm relatively still for a short period to minimize the flow of blood, and immediately notify a nurse, who can assist you in preventing **hematoma** formation. A hematoma occurs when blood forms under the skin due to insertion of a needle through a vein or artery, or in the case of fragile veins. To prevent accidental arterial puncture, do not select a vein that lies either over or close to an artery.

Selecting the perfect vein is not always easy. The patient may have only one arm available for use, and the skin on that arm may be sensitive to touch. In the event of dermatitis (inflammation of the skin in which the area is red and may contain skin lesions) or other conditions and when there are no other sites available, do not place the tourniquet directly on the arm. Instead, place the tourniquet over the patient's gown or clothing, or wrap the arm in gauze, then apply the tourniquet. It is also important that blood not be drawn from an extremity with an intravenous infusion (IV), because the contents of the infusion will alter the blood specimen results. In addition, for patients who have had a mastectomy (breast removal) or stroke, signs should be posted in the room that read, "NO BLOOD PRESSURES OR VENIPUNCTURES" in the affected arm.

1. If you accidentally hit an artery instead of a vein, how can you prevent a hematoma?

   _____

   _____

   _____

Common Veins Used for Phlebotomy

Phlebotomists must be familiar with the common arm veins used for phlebotomy. More sites for phlebotomy will be discussed later in this textbook. Such knowledge makes it easier to obtain blood specimens, even from patients with limited sites to access. The most commonly used veins for venipuncture are located in the middle of the arm and in front of the elbow. This area is called the **antecubital fossa,** and it is the site of the three most preferred veins for venipuncture (see Figure 2-8). The most commonly used vein for venipuncture is the **median cubital vein,** located in the middle of the forearm. The median cubital vein is the largest and best anchored or least moving vein in the forearm, making it the favored site for venipuncture. The next best site is the **cephalic vein,** which is also well anchored; however, it may be harder to palpate (feel). The third is the **basilic vein.** This site, though easier to palpate, is not well anchored, meaning it tends to roll when touched, making it more difficult to access. Additionally, the basilic vein lies close to the median nerve and the brachial artery, which must be avoided during venipuncture procedures. Other sites for venipuncture, such as veins in the back of the hand, are used when the antecubital veins are not accessible (see Figure 2-9). These hand veins are smaller, less anchored, and sometimes will require the use of a smaller needle. Using hand veins for venipuncture can also be more painful for the patient.

Figure 2-8 The veins in the arm most commonly used for venipuncture are located in the middle of the arm and in front of the elbow.

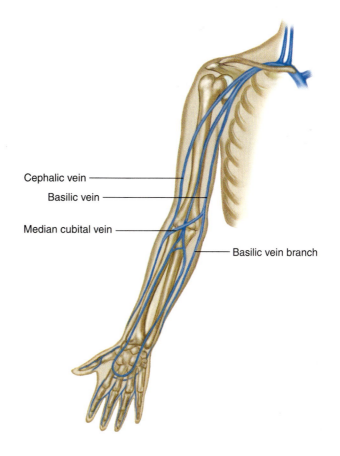

Cephalic vein

Basilic vein

Median cubital vein

Basilic vein branch

Figure 2-9 Veins in the back of the hand are sometimes used for venipuncture when the antecubital veins are not accessible.

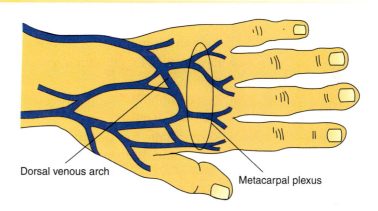

Dorsal venous arch

Metacarpal plexus

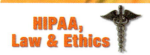

HIPAA, Law & Ethics

Selecting a Vein

The phlebotomist must use correct technique after properly selecting the vein. Accidental puncture of the median nerve could result in temporary or permanent loss of function of that arm. This would constitute an act of negligence, and there are cases in which patients have been awarded millions of dollars to compensate them for their losses. The best way to prevent injuring this nerve is to avoid "probing" around at the site.

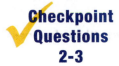
1. Name the types of vessels through which blood travels away from the heart and back to the heart.

   _____

   _____

   _____

   _____

2. Name three common veins in the antecubital fossa used for phlebotomy.

   _____

   _____

   _____

Answer the questions above and complete the *Blood Vessels* activity on the Student CD under Chapter 2 before you continue to the next section.

2-4 Blood and Blood Components

Blood is the transporting fluid of the body. Blood's composition is complex and essential to sustaining life. Blood has many important functions and also plays a role in other body functions, including the following:

- Responsible for transporting oxygen and nutrients to the cells and tissues of the body
- Responsible for transporting hormones to their target area, so that the body can function in its proper capacity
- Responsible for eliminating waste materials (excretion) from the body's cells
- Responsible for maintaining water balance for the cells and tissues of the body
- Responsible for transporting antibodies and protective substances throughout the body so they may attack infecting organisms and pathogens
- Assists with regulating body temperature
- Assists with maintaining acid-base balance

When a tube of blood is allowed to stand undisturbed, it will separate into two parts or components. One part is cellular (formed elements) and the other component is liquid (plasma).

Formed elements include your red blood cells (erythrocytes), white blood cells (leukocytes), and platelets (thrombocytes; see Figure 2-10). Formed elements make up about 45% of blood's total volume. Almost 99% of the circulating cells are red blood cells. Blood cells originate mostly from bone marrow (inside the bone). (See Table 2-1.) The liquid component or plasma is straw-colored or a pale yellow fluid that is comprised mostly of water. Plasma makes up about 55% of blood's total volume. Plasma contains 90% to 92% water and 8% to 10% solutes.

Figure 2-10   Formed elements of blood include white blood cells, red blood cells, and platelets.

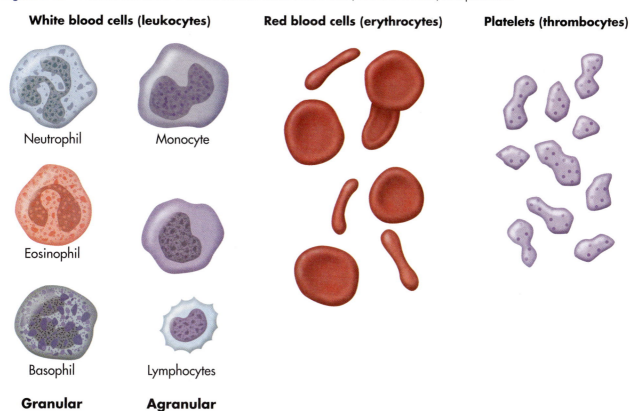

White blood cells (leukocytes)   **Red blood cells (erythrocytes)**   **Platelets (thrombocytes)**

Neutrophil   Monocyte

Eosinophil

Basophil   Lymphocytes

Granular   **Agranular**

TABLE 2-1   The Cellular Components of Blood

Blood Cells	Normal Quantity*	Description
Erythrocytes (red blood cells)	M. 4.5–6.2 million/mm³ F. 4.2–5.4 million/mm³	Contains hemoglobin; transports oxygen and carbon dioxide
Leukocytes (white blood cells)	5,000–10,000/mm³	Protects against infections
Thrombocytes (platelets)	150,000–450,000/mm³	Aids in blood clotting

*Blood cell ranges will vary according to lab reference materials.

Red Blood Cells (Erythrocytes)

Erythrocytes (red blood cells or RBCs) originate in the bone marrow and are the most numerous of all the blood cells. There are approximately 4.5 to 5 million red blood cells per cubic millimeter of blood, which means that about 18 million RBCs could sit on the head of a pin. Erythrocytes resemble the shape of a doughnut without a hole. This appearance is referred to as *biconcave* because both sides of the red blood cell cave inward at the center (see Figure 2-11). This shape allows flexibility, so that the RBCs can pass through the tiny capillaries.

Figure 2-11 **(a)** Red blood cells have a biconcave shape. **(b)** Scanning electron micrograph of red blood cells.

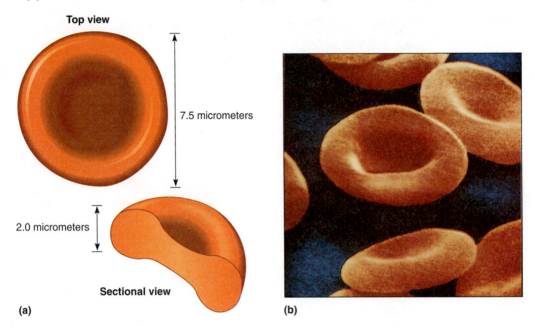

Top view

7.5 micrometers

2.0 micrometers

Sectional view

(a)

(b)

RBCs are responsible for the delivery of oxygen to, and removal of carbon dioxide from, every cell in the body, so they must be flexible enough to travel through the various sizes of blood vessels in order to perform their duty. Erythrocytes are constantly being manufactured by the bone marrow. The average life span of a red blood cell is about 120 days. After that they begin to fragment and rupture. The liver, spleen, and bone marrow will destroy old, worn-out red blood cells. There are thousands of red blood cells being formed and destroyed daily.

Red blood cells are responsible for carrying oxygen to every cell in the body and for removing carbon dioxide from the cells. This ability to transport oxygen and carbon dioxide occurs as a result of a very important molecule, called **hemoglobin.** Hemoglobin is made up of a protein molecule called *globin* and an iron compound called *heme.* A red blood cell contains several million molecules of hemoglobin. The normal adult hemoglobin ranges are as follows:

- Male = 14–18 grams/100 mL (1 deciliter) of blood
- Female = 12–16 grams/100 mL (1 deciliter) of blood

The presence of large amounts of oxygen attached to the hemoglobin in the red blood cells gives the blood a bright red color; this blood is referred to as oxygenated. When large amounts of carbon dioxide are attached to hemoglobin in the red blood cell, the color of the blood appears dark bluish-red, and the blood is considered deoxygenated.

Excessive blood loss, destruction of red blood cells, and/or decreased blood cell formation can all affect the supply of hemoglobin. An abnormally low hemoglobin level and/or decrease in the number of red blood cells is called anemia. Symptoms of anemia may include weakness, headache, difficulty breathing, and pale skin color. Conditions such as sickle cell anemia, hemophilia, forms of cancer, and a dietary deficiency of iron may all cause a decrease in hemoglobin and/or RBC numbers.

White Blood Cells (Leukocytes)

Leukocytes, or white blood cells, are not always confined to the vascular spaces to perform their duty. White blood cells are primarily responsible for destroying foreign substances such as pathogens (disease-producing microorganisms) and removing cellular debris. White blood cells can actually pass through the thin walls of capillaries to enter the tissues. This process is called **diapedesis,** and once white blood cells are at the site of foreign invaders, they can surround and destroy these pathogens through a process called **phagocytosis,** whereby the WBCs engulf or "eat" foreign substances and/or cellular debris.

Leukocytes are round and appear white because they lack hemoglobin. The average adult has between 5,000 and 10,000 white blood cells per cubic millimeter of blood, unless an infection is present. During a bacterial infection, the number of white blood cells increases in order to send an army of defender cells to the site of infection. Certain diseases such as leukemia cause an abnormally elevated number of white blood cells, and likewise there are conditions such as AIDS that cause a drastic decrease in the white blood cell count.

White blood cells are classified into two main categories, granulocytes and agranulocytes, depending on the presence or absence of small particles in the **cytoplasm** (area of the cell outside the nucleus) known as granules. If granules are present in the cytoplasm, they are referred to as granulocytes, and if no granules are present, they are called agranulocytes. Table 2-2 presents descriptions of the various types of granulocytes (neutrophils, basophils, and eosinophils) and agranulocytes (monocytes and lymphocytes). A special test known as a differential uses Wright's stain to differentiate between granulocytes and agranulocytes.

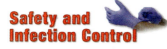

Safety and Infection Control

Immunocompromised Patients

The phlebotomist may be required to draw blood from patients who are immunocompromised. One such situation is when the patient has an abnormally low neutrophil count and therefore has a low resistance to infections. Even the slightest infection can prove to be life-threatening to these patients. In addition to Standard Precautions, immunocompromised patients require extra measures to be taken in order to prevent transmission of pathogens. The phlebotomist must perform hand hygiene and apply sterile personal protective equipment, not only to protect him- or herself but to protect the patient. Meticulous hand hygiene and not entering the patient's room if the common cold or other symptoms of illness are present are a must to prevent severe illness and even death in patients with low resistance to infections.

The most numerous of all the white blood cells are the **neutrophils.** The granules in the cytoplasm of neutrophils appear lavender when stained. Neutrophils are the main warriors against infections, and their average life span is from 6 hours to a few days. They move quickly to the site of infection and engulf the invader. Following the battle between neutrophils and

TABLE 2-2 Types of White Blood Cells

Type		% of Total WBC Count	Description
Granulocytes			
	Neutrophils have distinct nuclei with many lobes.	60%–70%	Aid in phagocytosis; release pyrogens to cause fever; use lysosomal enzymes to phagocytize bacteria (stain lavender or pink)
	Eosinophils have cytoplasmic granules that stain red.	1%–4%	Assist with inflammatory responses; secrete chemicals that destroy certain parasites; level increases with allergies and parasitic infection (stain red-orange)
	Basophils have cytoplasmic granules that stain deep blue.	0%–1%	Assist with inflammatory response by releasing histamine; release heparin (anticoagulant) and produce a vasodilator; count increases with chronic inflammation and during healing from infection (stain dark blue or blue-black)
Agranulocytes			
	Monocytes have large kidney-shaped nuclei. They do not have cytoplasmic granules.	2%–6%	Largest WBCs; carry out phagocytosis; effective against chronic infections such as tuberculosis (TB)
	Lymphocytes have large round nuclei.	20%–30%	Assist immune system by producing antibodies; level increases during viral infections

pathogens, **pus** is formed, which contains the remaining dead neutrophils, pathogens, and parts of the cells at the site of infection or injury.

The second type of granulocytes are the **eosinophils.** These white blood cells are present in a very small quantity. The cytoplasmic granules stain bright red-orange in color with Eosin. These granulocytes also assist with inflammatory reactions to prevent spread of inflammation. As a matter of fact, during parasitic infections with pinworms, eosinophils secrete chemicals that can destroy the parasite. Eosinophils actually ingest and destroy foreign proteins, a process known as phagocytosis. They live for about 8 to 12 days and increase in number in response to parasitic infections and allergic conditions.

Basophils are the least common granulocytes, and the cytoplasmic granules stain dark blue or blue-black with basic dyes. These white blood cells assist with the inflammatory response, which is local swelling in response to injury or a foreign invader. Basophils release histamine, which is a substance that causes capillary walls to dilate, allowing blood to enter the infected site. In addition to histamine, basophils also release heparin, which is an **anticoagulant.** Body areas containing large amounts of blood, such as the liver and lungs, have the largest amount of basophils, so it is believed that the release of heparin in these areas prevents the formation of tiny blood clots.

Agranulocytes, named because their cytoplasm contains no granules, include monocytes and lymphocytes. **Monocytes** are the largest of all agranular white blood cells. Their primary function is phagocytosis. Monocytes are not present in large amounts, but they survive for several months. Monocytes are effective against chronic infections. They are capable of leaving the bloodstream to move into the tissues. When they do this they are referred to as "macrophages." These macrophages are larger cells, and they not only engulf pathogens, but they also remove old, worn-out red blood cells when performing their phagocytic actions.

Lymphocytes are also agranulocytes, and they play an important role in the body's immune system. They produce **antibodies** and other chemicals that destroy pathogens. Lymphocytes can be divided into two groups: T-lymphocytes and B-lymphocytes. T-lymphocytes are responsible for mediating cell-mediated immune responses. T-lymphocytes can further be subdivided into Helper T cells or Suppressor T cells. (Helper T cells or CD4 + cells are those that are destroyed by the Human Immunodeficiency Virus or HIV.) T cells are formed in the thymus, while B cells are formed in the bone marrow and lymph nodes. The life span of lymphocytes ranges from a few days to several years. B cells help defend the body by synthesizing and releasing antibody molecules. The antibodies are made to specifically match the antigens that triggered their production. Other cells of the immune system, such as natural killer (NK) cells or macrophages have functions such as destruction of cancer cells or direct engulfment of foreign substances. The production of antibodies by plasma cells (antibody-producing cells arising from B-lymphocytes) is called the humoral response. That is because the immunity is in the humors or fluids of the body. This is also called antibody-mediated immunity. T-lympocytes are involved in cell-mediated immunity.

During instances of suspected infection, it is very helpful for the physician to know the percentages of each type of white blood cell to assist with diagnosing and treating the patient. This blood test is called a differential, and it can identify quantities of each of the cellular components using only one tube of blood. Differentials will be discussed further in Chapter 5.

Platelets (Thrombocytes)

Thrombocytes, or platelets, are the smallest in size of all the cellular components. The life span of platelets is about 9 to 12 days, and the normal adult range is between 150,000 and 450,000 per cubic millimeter of blood. Unlike the other blood cells, platelets are not complete cells; instead they are fragments from a larger cell found in bone marrow. Platelets are instrumental in preventing blood loss because when an injury occurs, they are the first cells to arrive at the site. Bleeding is diminished or halted as a result of platelets sticking to the site of injury and forming a platelet plug. Platelets also secrete a substance serotin, which causes the blood vessels to spasm or narrow and decrease blood loss until the clot forms. Platelets, along with substances in the liquid composition of blood, are essential for minimizing blood loss as a result of injury. Platelets are formed in the bone marrow and old platelets are trapped by the spleen.

Liquid Component (Plasma)

The liquid portion of whole blood is called **plasma,** which is a pale yellow fluid comprised mostly of water. Constituents of plasma include the following:

- *Water* is 90% to 92% of plasma. This percentage is monitored by the kidneys and the pituitary gland. It is affected by the large intestine and the amount of water consumed.
- *Nutrients* are materials passed through the digestive system directly into the bloodstream. These include things such as cholesterols, fatty acids, amino acids, and glucose.
- *Hormones* assist with chemical reactions and allow the body to maintain a constant balance. One example is thymosin, which helps the immune system battle foreign invaders. A more common hormone is insulin, which regulates the amount of sugar in the bloodstream.
- *Electrolytes* include sodium, potassium, calcium, magnesium, and chloride. These are found in food and chemical processes.
- *Proteins* such as fibrinogen, globulin, and albumin:
  - *Fibrinogen* is a protein that aids in clotting and is manufactured in the liver. (If this clotting factor was missing from plasma, the remaining liquid would be referred to as **serum.**)
  - *Globulin* is manufactured in the lymphatic system and the liver. It helps with the production of antibodies, which fight foreign invaders within the body.
  - *Albumin* is the most abundant of all plasma proteins. It is a product of the liver, and it helps to pull water into the bloodstream to assist in regulating blood pressure.
- *Waste* is produced as a result of the body's cells undergoing a chemical reaction. Plasma is responsible for carrying waste to the organs responsible for getting rid of or excreting it. Examples of waste products include urea, uric acid, creatinine, and xanthine.
- *Protective substances* include antitoxins, opsonins, agglutinin, bacteriolysins, hypoxanthine, adenine, and carnine.

Plasma and serum have a distinct difference. Plasma is the liquid portion of *unclotted* blood, collected in a tube with an anticoagulant that

Figure 2-12 Centrifuged blood sample and peripheral blood smear showing blood components.

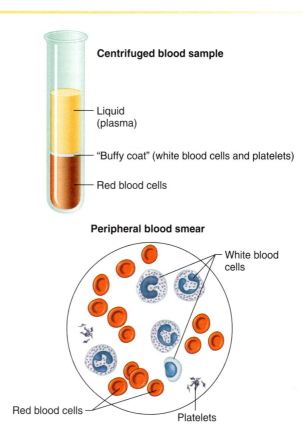

Centrifuged blood sample

— Liquid (plasma)

— "Buffy coat" (white blood cells and platelets)

— Red blood cells

Peripheral blood smear

White blood cells

Red blood cells

Platelets

prevents clotting. The most commonly used tubes have purple or lavender tops. Serum is the liquid portion of *clotted* blood, collected in a tube without an anticoagulant, in which the clot has been allowed to form. The clot forms in serum when fibrinogen converts into fibrin and traps formed elements of the blood. When the clot forms, the clotting factors are depleted and the resultant fluid is known as serum. This process of clotting is called **coagulation.** When laboratory tubes contain an anticoagulant that prevents the clotting of blood, it can be separated into cells and plasma by **centrifugation.** The results of centrifugation are shown in Figure 2-12. Centrifugation will be discussed further in Chapter 5.

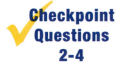

Checkpoint Questions 2-4

1. What type of blood cells have hemoglobin and what is hemoglobin's purpose?

_____

_____

_____

_____

2. What is the major function of leukocytes?

_____

_____

_____

3. What is the difference between serum and plasma?

_____

_____

_____

_____

Answer the questions above and complete the *Blood and Blood Components* activity on the Student CD under Chapter 2 before you continue to the next section.

2-5 Hemostasis and Blood Coagulation

It is important for the phlebotomist to understand how bleeding is controlled naturally. Both venipuncture and dermal puncture create injuries to the blood vessels, and the body's natural defenses must stop the bleeding. The medical term **hemostasis** breaks down into *hemo,* meaning "blood," and *stasis,* meaning "stopping." Following an injury there are four major events involved in stopping the flow of blood at the injured site:

1. blood vessel spasm (vasoconstriction)
2. platelet plug formation
3. blood clotting (coagulation)
4. fibrinolysis or dissolving of the clot and return of the vessel to normal function

Figure 2-13 illustrates these four events.

Blood Vessel Spasm

If the blood vessel is small and the injury is limited, a blood vessel spasm alone may stop the bleeding. At the time of injury, the involved blood vessels will constrict (decrease in diameter or size), and this decreases the amount of blood flowing through the vessel and consequently stops or controls bleeding.

Platelet Plug Formation

In the event bleeding continues in spite of the blood vessel spasms, platelets are then called into action. The torn, inner lining of the blood vessels releases chemical signals, which stimulate the arrival of several platelets at the site of injury. These platelets clump together to form a platelet plug, which further decreases the flow of blood from the injured site. This process occurs within seconds after an injury and is known as primary hemostasis.

Blood Clotting

Extensive injury to larger blood vessels will generally require all three steps in the hemostasis process. The last step is coagulation, or blood clotting,

Figure 2-13   Events of hemostasis.

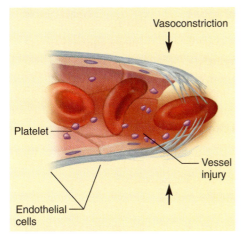

Vasoconstriction

Platelet

Vessel injury

Endothelial cells

(1) Blood vessel spasm

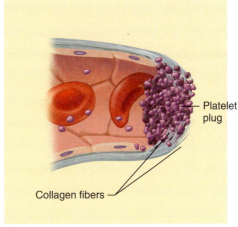

Platelet plug

Collagen fibers

(2) Platelet plug formation

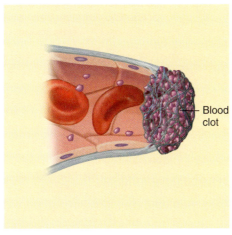

Blood clot

(3) Blood clotting

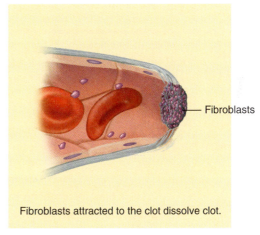

Fibroblasts

Fibroblasts attracted to the clot dissolve clot.

(4) Fibrinolysis

which requires the presence of specific clotting factors to form a blood clot. At the time of injury to the blood vessel, certain inactive clotting chemicals are called into action. These clotting factors come together through a complex series of events, and the end product is **thrombin,** which is an enzyme used to convert the plasma protein fibrinogen into **fibrin.** Once fibrin has been produced, the threadlike composition of fibrin forms a net or meshlike sac that adheres to the site of injury, trapping blood cells and other particles to form a clot. This process takes several minutes and is known as secondary hemostasis.

Fibrinolysis

The clot attracts and stimulates the growth of fibroblasts and smooth muscle cells within the vessel wall. This begins the repair process, which ultimately results in the dissolution of the clot or fibrinolysis and return of the vessel to normal.

Lack of Clotting Factors

Not all individuals possess the natural clotting factors. Some people are born with medical conditions that cause bleeding disorders; an example is hemophilia. Persons taking anticoagulants (e.g., heparin and coumadin) or those lacking natural clotting ability require close monitoring following venipuncture. The phlebotomist must apply manual pressure to the site for a minimum of three to five minutes to ensure that bleeding has stopped.

1. You have just completed a venipuncture on a patient who is taking coumadin. When you lift the gauze to check the site, it continues to bleed heavily. What should you do?

   _____

   _____

Checkpoint Question 2-5

1. List in order the four events involved in stopping the flow of blood at an injured site.

   _____

   _____

   _____

   _____

 Answer the question above and complete the *Hemostasis and Blood Coagulation* activity on the Student CD under Chapter 2 before you continue to the next section.

2-6 ABO and Rh Blood Types

If 20 tubes of blood were lined up on a counter in the laboratory, they all would look very much alike even though they are very different. The naked eye is not capable of detecting the inherited identifying structures on the surface of individual red blood cells, known as **antigens.**

The ABO blood group consists of four different **blood types:** A, B, AB, and O. They are distinguished from each other in part by their antigens and antibodies (see Figure 2-14).

Agglutination is the clumping of red blood cells following a blood transfusion. This clumping is not desirable because it leads to red blood cell destruction, which leads to anemia or a transfusion reaction that can be deadly. Agglutination occurs because proteins called *antigens* on the surface of red blood cells bind to *antibodies* in plasma. To prevent agglutination, antigens should not be mixed with antibodies that will bind to them. Fortunately, most antibodies do not bind to antigens on blood cells; only very specific ones bind to them.

Figure 2-14 A, B, AB, and O blood types.

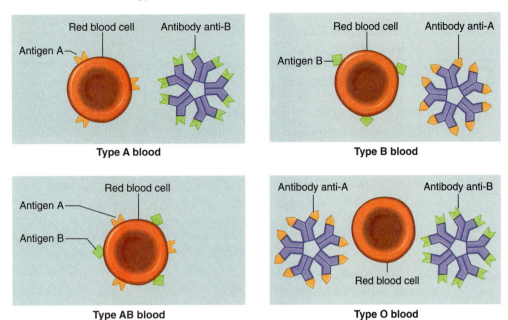

Type A

People with type A blood have antigen A on the surface of their red blood cells. They also have antibody B in their plasma. Antibody B will only bind to antigen B.

Type B

People with type B blood have antigen B on the surface of their red blood cells. They also have antibody A in their plasma. If a person with type A blood is given type B blood, then the antibody B in the recipient's blood will bind with the red blood cells of the donor blood because those cells have antigen B on their surfaces. Therefore, agglutination occurs, and the donated red blood cells are destroyed. This is why a person with type A blood should not be given type B blood (and vice versa).

Type AB

People with type AB blood have both antigen A and antigen B on the surface of their red blood cells. They have neither antibody A nor antibody B in their plasma. People with type AB blood are called universal recipients, because most of them can receive all ABO blood types. They can receive these blood types because they lack antibody A and antibody B in their plasma, so there is no reaction with antigens A and B of the donor blood.

Type O

People with type O blood have neither antigen A nor antigen B on the surface of their red blood cells. However, they do have both antibody A and antibody B in their plasma. People with type O blood are called universal donors because their blood can be given to most people regardless of recipients' blood type. Type O blood will not agglutinate when given to other people because it does not have the antigens to bind to antibody A or antibody B.

The Rh Factor

The **Rh antigen** is a protein that was first discovered on red blood cells of the Rhesus monkey, hence the name Rh. People who are Rh-positive have red blood cells that contain the Rh antigen. People who are Rh-negative have red blood cells that do not contain the Rh antigen. If a person who is Rh-negative is given Rh-positive blood, then the Rh-negative person's blood will make antibodies that bind to the Rh antigens. If the Rh-negative person is given Rh-positive blood a second time, the antibodies will bind to the donor cells and agglutination will occur.

Clinically, it is very important for a female to know her Rh type. If an Rh-negative female mates with an Rh-positive male, there is a 50-50 chance that her fetus will be Rh-positive. After birth when the blood of an Rh-positive fetus mixes with the blood of a mother who is Rh-negative, the mother develops antibodies against the fetus's red blood cells. The first Rh-positive fetus usually does not suffer from these antibodies because mother's body has not yet generated the antibodies. However, if the mother conceives another Rh-positive fetus, the fetus's blood will be attacked by the antibodies right away. The fetus then develops a condition called *erythroblastosis fetalis,* and the baby is born severely anemic, often needing multiple blood transfusions at birth and often several times as a neonate. Without treatment, the baby may die before birth or after delivery. Erythroblastosis fetalis is prevented by giving an Rh-negative woman the drug RhoGAM®. RhoGAM® prevents an Rh-negative mother from making antibodies against the Rh antigen. Blood tests such as the direct Coombs and bilirubin may be ordered to evaluate the newborn for any blood incompatibility between the mother and newborn.

Transfusion Reactions

Hemolytic transfusion reactions occur when agglutination occurs from a transfusion. Transfusion reactions can range from mild, which may produce a slight fever or hives, to severe, resulting in death. To avoid reactions patients are given type-specific blood or blood products even in emergencies. Phlebotomists are frequently asked to draw blood for typing and cross-matching patients prior to the patient receiving blood and blood products. To prevent transfusion reactions you must always use two patient identifiers and label the blood and blood products accurately. An incorrectly labeled type and cross-match specimen could cause a patient to die.

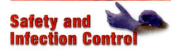

Safety and Infection Control

Type and Cross-Match Blood Specimens

For most blood tests, phlebotomists must simply initial the tube and requisition form. However, more complete identification is usually required on both the specimen tube and requisition form for all "type and cross-match" orders. This may include a signature, ID (identification) number, or barcoding of armband and specimen labels. Follow the policy at the facility where you are employed.

Some individuals elect to have their own blood drawn at outpatient settings so it can be stored in a blood bank for later use if they should need it. When this predrawn, donated blood is given back to the patient, it is referred to as an autologous blood transfusion. During surgical procedures where extensive blood may be lost, patients can be readministered some of the blood lost during the surgery, and this would still be considered an autologous blood transfusion.

Troubleshooting Blood Suppliers

Many agencies such as the American Red Cross, United Blood Services, and Life Share collect and supply blood. All agencies typically have specific criteria for blood donors.

The American Red Cross states that a donor:

- Must be at least 17 years old
- Must be in good general health
- Must weigh at least 110 pounds

1. What qualities should blood donors have?

_____

_____

Checkpoint Questions 2-6

1. What are two ways a phlebotomist can prevent a transfusion reaction?

_____

_____

_____

_____

2. Why is blood typically typed and cross-matched before a transfusion?

_____

_____

_____

 Answer the questions above and complete the *ABO and Rh Blood Types* activity on the Student CD under Chapter 2 before you continue to the next section.

Chapter Summary

- The vascular system consists of a network of vessels and, along with the heart, provide for circulation of the blood.
- Coronary circulation provides blood to the heart. Systemic circulation provides blood to and from the body. Blood travels to and from the lungs and obtains oxygen and removes carbon dioxide from the blood.
- Blood vessel layers include the tunica intima (innermost), tunica media (middle), and tunica adventitia (outermost).
- All arteries, with the exception of the pulmonary artery, carry oxygenated blood to the body. All veins, with the exception of the pulmonary artery, carry deoxygenated blood back to the heart and lungs. Arterioles are small arteries and venules are small veins. Capillaries provide a link between arterioles and venules and allow for gas exchange.
- The three veins most commonly used for phlebotomy are located in the antecubital fossa. They include the median cubital, cephalic, and basilic veins.
- Blood is responsible for transporting oxygen and nutrients to the cells and tissues of the body, transporting hormones to their target area, eliminating waste materials (excretion) from the body's cells, maintaining water balance for the cells and tissues of the body, and transporting antibodies and protective substances.
- The major components of blood include formed elements (erythrocytes, leukocytes, and platelets) and plasma.
- Red blood cells transport oxygen and carbon dioxide. White blood cells destroy foreign invaders and remove cellular debris. Platelets are essential for clotting.
- Granular white blood cells include neutrophils for phagocytosis, eosinophils for phagocytosis, and basophils for release of histamine and heparin. Agranulocytes include monocytes that fight chronic infections and lymphocytes that assist the immune system in producing antibodies.
- Plasma is the liquid portion of unclotted blood. Serum is the liquid portion of blood collected in a tube without anticoagulant.
- Hemostasis or stopping of blood includes four major events: blood vessel spasm, platelet plug formation, blood clotting, and fibrinolysis.
- ABO and Rh blood types are determined by the type of antigen found on the red blood cells.

Chapter Review

Label the Figure

Using the diagram provided, place the correct letter next to the correct structure.

basilic

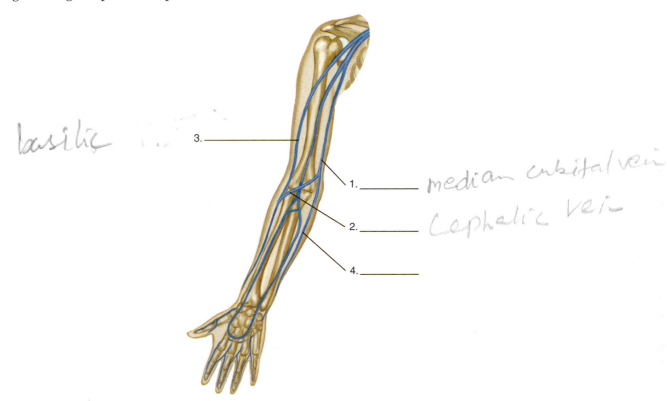

3. _____

1. _____ median cubital vein

2. _____ cephalic vein

4. _____

a. basilic vein.

b. cephalic vein.

c. median cubital vein.

d. basilic vein branch.

Matching

Match the following terms with their correct description or definition:

_____ **5.** oxygenated

_____ **6.** deoxygenated

_____ **7.** artery

_____ **8.** vein

a. Carries deoxygenated blood away from the heart.

b. A very small vein.

c. A very small artery.

d. Blood with high oxygen concentration.

e. Largest vein in the body.

_____ 9. venule

_____ 10. arteriole

_____ 11. aorta

_____ 12. vena cava

_____ 13. capillary

_____ 14. tunica intima

_____ 15. tunica media

_____ 16. tunica adventitia

_____ 17. serum

_____ 18. plasma

_____ 19. pulmonary artery

_____ 20. pulmonary vein

f. Smallest blood vessel in the body.

g. Carries oxygenated blood to the heart.

h. Largest artery in the body.

i. Middle layer of blood vessels.

j. Blood with high carbon dioxide concentration.

k. Contains fibrinogen.

l. Blood vessel that carries blood from the heart.

m. Outer covering of the blood vessels.

n. Blood vessel that carries blood toward the heart.

o. Innermost smooth layer of the blood vessels.

p. Fluid left after blood has clotted.

True or False

Write T or F in the blank to indicate whether you think the statement is true or false. Correct any false statements to make them true.

_____ 21. Arteries contain valves to prevent the backflow of blood.

_____ 22. At any point in time about 70% of your blood is stored in your veins.

_____ 23. Venous blood is a dark red color.

_____ 24. Arterial blood is a bright red color.

_____ 25. The median cubital vein is the preferred site for venipuncture.

_____ 26. There are approximately 100,000 miles of blood vessels in the vascular system.

_____ 27. Arteries are the smallest of the vessel family and their primary function is to carry deoxygenated blood to the heart.

_____ 28. Pulmonary circulation consists of oxygenated blood leaving the lungs and heading to all the systems of the body.

_____ 29. Blood is composed of two major parts (plasma and formed elements).

_____ 30. A hematoma occurs when blood pools form under the skin due to insertion of a needle through a vein or artery, or in the case of fragile veins.

Matching

Match each blood component with the correct description by writing the appropriate letter in the space provided.

_____ 31. lymphocytes

_____ 32. monocytes

_____ 33. diapedesis

a. Performs phagocytosis to destroy pathogens.

b. Smallest of all the blood components; considered to be a cell fragment.

c. The most numerous of the WBCs.

_____ 34. eosinophils

_____ 35. erythrocytes

_____ 36. leukocytes

_____ 37. neutrophils

_____ 38. basophils

_____ 39. platelets

d. Process by which WBCs pass through the capillary walls to fight pathogens.

e. The least common granulocyte.

f. The largest of all WBCs.

g. Contains hemoglobin and transports oxygen and carbon dioxide.

h. Produces antibodies that help destroy pathogens.

i. Assists with inflammatory processes; level is elevated in the presence of allergies and parasites.

Ordering

Put the events of hemostasis (coagulation) in the correct order from 1 to 4.

_____ 40. Formation of the platelet plug

_____ 41. Blood vessel spasm

_____ 42. Blood clotting

_____ 43. Fibrinolysis

Fill in the Blanks

Write the appropriate word or letter to complete the sentence correctly.

44. _____(s) are located on the surface of the RBCs.

45. The liquid portion of the blood is referred to as _____ or plasma.

46. _____(s) are present in the blood plasma.

47. Persons with type _____ blood have the A antigens on the surface of their red blood cells.

48. Type _____ blood does not contain A or B antigens.

What Should You Do?

Use your critical thinking skills to respond to the following situations.

49. A phlebotomist is attempting to obtain blood from an unconscious patient. When the needle is inserted into the arm, the phlebotomist observes a bright red, pulsating flow of blood entering the syringe. What may have occurred, and what should the phlebotomist do next?

_____

_____

50. An immunocompromised patient requires routine blood to be drawn and the phlebotomist has just received a STAT page that needs to be done immediately. Should the phlebotomist proceed into the room quickly and just draw this patient's blood, or should the phlebotomist come back at a later time if there is no one else available to draw the blood for him or her? Give an explanation for your response.

_____

_____

51. A patient exposed to a parasitic infection may experience elevated WBCs. What type of WBC will increase in number during an infection of this type?

_____

_____

52. Lymphocytes play an important role in the body's immune system. They produce antibodies and other chemicals that destroy pathogens. What are the two types of lymphocytes that play an effective role in the body's immune system?

_____

_____

53. Platelets are responsible for clotting blood. When a blood vessel is damaged, the vessel collagen fibers come in contact with the platelets. The platelets produce a sticky substance allowing them to stick to the collagen fibers. What would happen to a patient who is experiencing a low platelet count? How would you collect blood from a patient with a low platelet count?

_____

_____

Get Connected *Internet Activity*

Visit the McGraw-Hill Higher Education Online Learning Center *Phlebotomy for Health Care Personnel* Website at **www.mhhe.com/healthcareskills** to complete the following activity.

Take a virtual field trip to the MedlinePlus Internet site to learn more about circulation and the blood. Research the site to complete these activities.
1. Create a picture collage or bulletin board demonstrating circulation or the process of hemostasis.
2. Develop a presentation about the components of blood or the ABO and Rh blood systems.

Using the Student CD

Now that you have completed the material in the chapter text, return to the Student CD and complete any chapter activities you have not yet done. Practice your terminology with the "Key Term Concentration" game. Review the chapter material with the "Spin the Wheel" game. Take the final chapter test and complete the troubleshooting question. E-mail or print your results to document your proficiency for this chapter.

Equipment for Specimen Collection

3

Learning Outcomes

Upon completion of this chapter, you should be able to:

- List the information required on a requisition form.
- Describe computer use in phlebotomy.
- Describe the supplies and general equipment required for phlebotomy.
- Describe the components of the evacuated tube system.
- Explain the proper method for needle disposal.
- Identify the type, explain the mechanism of action, and identify the evacuated tube color associated with each additive.
- Explain the order of draw for evacuated tubes.
- List the components of the butterfly infusion and syringe systems.
- Identify the equipment needed to perform dermal puncture.

Key Terms

additive	evacuated collection tube
aerosol	evacuated tube holder
antiglycolytic	gauge
antiseptic	hemolysis
bacteriostatic	microsample
bevel	requisition
butterfly needle set	sterile
capillary action	syringe
centrifuge	tourniquet
dermal	winged set

3-1 Introduction

The phlebotomist must be familiar with the process and all the tools that are involved in venipuncture and dermal puncture procedures. This includes the various pieces of equipment used for the different methods of blood collection. In addition, the phlebotomist should know the ordering process, including paper or computer work that must be completed prior to blood collection. A proper blood collection procedure starts with the order, documents, and appropriate equipment. The actual collection of blood must be done in the correct order.

Checkpoint Question 3-1

1. What does the phlebotomist need to know prior to the blood collection procedure?

_____

_____

_____

_____

3-2 Laboratory Requisitions

The phlebotomy procedure begins when a physician or other qualified health care practitioner orders that a blood test be performed on a patient. The order indicates that a test **requisition** be completed, or the health care practitioner generates a requisition. (A requisition is a hard copy documentation of the blood test ordered.) In some cases, the physician may request a blood test over the telephone or through the computer. Clerical personnel, nurses, or even a phlebotomist may fill out the requisition form per a physician's request. Regardless of how the order is received, a written or computer-generated requisition form must be completed. Computer requisitions usually contain the actual labels that are to be placed on the specimens once they have been collected. Although used infrequently, there are also various types of handwritten requisition forms available (Figure 3-1). Some

Figure 3-1 For the phlebotomist to perform blood collection, a requisition form must be completed with: **(a)** patient's name; **(b)** requesting physician; **(c)** medical record number; **(d)** date and time requested; **(e)** date and time performed; **(f)** test to be performed; **(g)** test status; **(h)** patient location; and **(i)** phlebotomist initials.

	TEST	INSTRUCTIONS	RESULTS	PERFORMED BY
	Blood glucose	Fasting		

HARBOR HOSPITAL
Department of Laboratory Medicine

DATE REQUESTED 5/22/XXXX   TIME REQUESTED 9:15/AM
DATE COLLECTED 5/22/XXXX   TIME COLLECTED 9:30/AM — (e)

NAME Dee Preston — (a)

ADDRESS 99 College Blvd.
Happy, VA

PATIENT ROOM NO. 199   BED NO. 3 — (h)

AGE 35   SEX M   HOSPITAL I.D. NO. 86123 — (c)

PHYSICIAN Dr. Adams — (b)

TODAY ☒   ROUTINE ☐

EMERGENCY ☐   SIGNED ℒℱ — (i)

Figure 3-2 An electronic requisition form like this one may be used at the facility where you are employed.

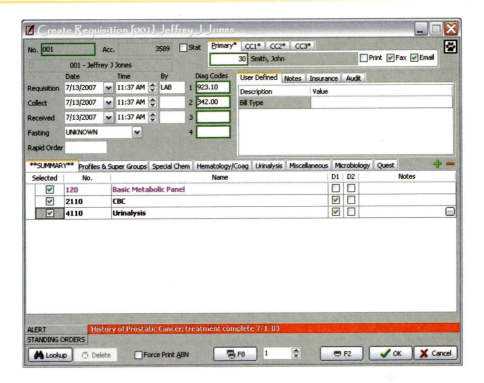

laboratories require separate requisitions for each department, which may be color-coded or numbered to identify the laboratory to which the specimen will be transported for analysis. No matter what type of requisition form is used, the phlebotomist must be able to read and interpret it quickly and accurately.

Patient Education & Communication

Computers in the Laboratory

In many health care facilities, when a laboratory test is ordered it is entered in a computer at the patient care station or even by the physician in his office. The computer in the laboratory receives the order and prints the requisition for the phlebotomist to take to the patient (see Figure 3-2). Very specialized "laboratory information systems" are also found in clinical laboratory facilities that connect to the laboratory analyzers and remote locations, plus provide security for patient data in order to comply with HIPAA. Essentially, in these interconnected systems all patient data, orders, results, and patient charges are kept in one system.

It is the responsibility of the phlebotomist to examine all requisitions carefully prior to leaving the laboratory to collect the specimen or drawing blood from a patient. All requisitions must contain certain basic information to ensure that the specimen drawn and the test results reported are for the correct patient. In special testing conditions, such as when the patient is required to fast (no food or liquids except water) prior to the draw or when blood must be drawn at an exact time, these requirements should be included on the requisition form. The requisition should include the following information:

- Patient's name
- Date of birth (as recommended by your institution and/or no medical record number is available)
- Ordering physician's name
- Patient's medical record number
- Date and time the test is to be performed
- Type of test to be performed
- Test status (timed, fasting, STAT, ASAP, etc.)
- Patient's location (if inpatient)
- Social Security number (if recommended by your institution)
- Initials of phlebotomist

It is not uncommon for the phlebotomist to find a discrepancy in the spelling of the patient's name on the lab requisition form when comparing it to the patient's wrist (identification) band. It is the phlebotomist's responsibility to find out which spelling of the patient's name is correct before collecting specimens. Make sure the correct spelling is on the requisition form, the ID band, and the specimen(s), once labeled.

Troubleshooting Patient Identification

In the event of two spellings for the same last name, such as *Stevenson* and *Stephenson,* the phlebotomist must determine the correct spelling *prior* to obtaining the blood specimen. Also check at least one other identifier such as date of birth and/or medical record number.

Question: The requisition form indicates the patient's name is John M. Smith, but when you check the identification band it shows "John N. Smyth." What should you do?

_____

_____

Checkpoint Questions 3-2

1. What data is included on a patient requisition?

_____

_____

_____

2. How are computers used in the laboratory?

_____

_____

_____

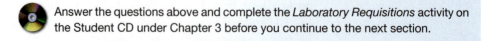

Answer the questions above and complete the *Laboratory Requisitions* activity on the Student CD under Chapter 3 before you continue to the next section.

3-3 Specimen Collection Equipment

Most blood tests require collection of a blood specimen by venipuncture. This process is often referred to as "drawing blood." To prepare for a routine venipuncture, the phlebotomist must assemble all the equipment and supplies used in the process (see Figure 3-3):

- Gloves
- Tourniquet
- Alcohol prep pads
- Gauze pads
- Adhesive bandage or tape
- Needles
- Evacuated tube holder or syringe
- Sharps (needle disposal) container
- Permanent marker, pen, or computer labels
- Evacuated tubes

Gloves

Gloves are available in a variety of materials and in many sizes and styles. Gloves may be non-powdered latex or non-latex. Nitrile, synthetic vinyl, or other non-latex gloves are used frequently and for persons who are sensitive to latex products. Latex gloves should not be used when a patient has latex allergies. Nonsterile gloves are acceptable for blood collection because the procedure is not a sterile procedure such as surgery. Powder in many gloves can become a contaminant in or on the specimen; therefore powder-free gloves are recommended. OSHA regulations require that gloves be worn during the phlebotomy procedure and changed after each patient. Proper fit is important for safety. If too small, they may tear. If too large, items may be

Figure 3-3 A variety of equipment is needed to perform a routine venipuncture.

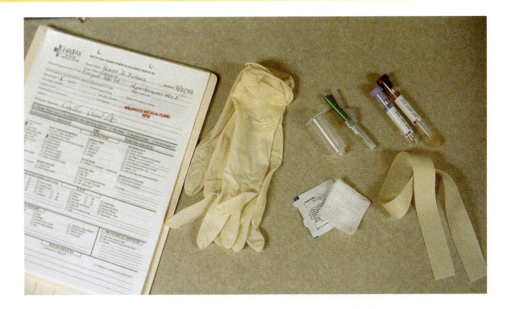

dropped (see Figure 3-4). Replace gloves immediately when ripped, torn, or contaminated. Remember during blood collection to always wash your hands or perform hand hygiene before applying and after removing the gloves.

Adherence to the gloving protocol is essential to prevent transmission of bloodborne pathogens; however, a large number of health care workers experience severe allergies as a result of wearing latex gloves. Classic signs of latex allergy are itchy, red hands following the removal of latex gloves. Handwashing immediately following the removal of latex gloves decreases the time of exposure and prevents transmission of the latex to other body areas such as the eyes and mucous membranes. Latex allergies are not to be taken lightly. Severe allergic reactions and even death have resulted from latex allergies. If latex allergy is suspected, the phlebotomist may consider undergoing specialized immunologic evaluations such as skin tests and blood testing. Avoiding latex gloves or other latex equipment is essential. Health care facilities are required by law to provide latex-free gloves for health care employees with latex allergies. Glove liners are available but only used for long-term glove use such as specimen processing. Glove liners make it difficult to palpate veins. Wearing well-fitting, non-latex gloves is the best policy for the phlebotomist.

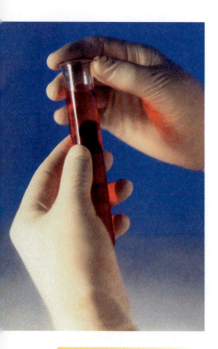

Figure 3-4 Well-fitting gloves must be worn during phlebotomy procedures.

Tourniquet

A **tourniquet** is a length of rubber tubing that is wrapped around the arm to slow down the flow of venous blood, causing a backup of blood and increased pressure. Tourniquets are used during venipuncture to make it easier to locate a patient's veins. When a tourniquet is applied to an arm, the veins become enlarged, making them easier to find and penetrate with a needle. Several styles of tourniquets are available. Each phlebotomist must decide his or her preference. Common types are rubber tubes, thin rubber bands, or strips of elastic fabric (see Figure 3-5). Non-latex tourniquets are preferred to avoid any chance of developing a latex allergy. Sometimes a blood pressure cuff is used to help locate an appropriate site for venipuncture in people with veins that are difficult to "feel" or "see." When using a blood pressure cuff, the cuff should be inflated to a pressure between the systolic and diastolic pressure. Whatever type of regular tourniquet is used, it must be disposed of after the procedure or used again only on the same patient if not visibly contaminated. For example, when a patient at an inpatient

Figure 3-5 Tourniquets are used to slow the blood and make venipuncture easier. They come in a variety of types.

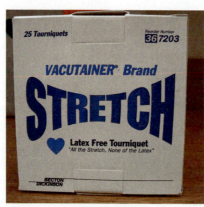

(a) Non-latex tourniquet box

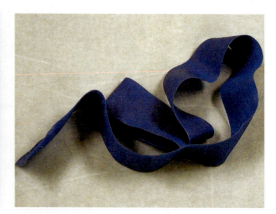

(b) Single tourniquet

facility requires multiple blood collections, a tourniquet may be kept at the bedside and reused only if it is not contaminated. Tourniquets should *not* be cleaned and reused. The tourniquet should not be left on the arm longer than one minute at a time. Leaving the tourniquet on too long can actually change the results of certain blood tests. If it takes longer than one minute to complete the procedure, loosen the tourniquet for at least one minute. After one minute the tourniquet can be reapplied.

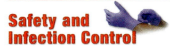

Safety and Infection Control

Latex Allergies and Phlebotomy

Natural rubber latex (NRL) comes from a liquid in tropical rubber trees. It is frequently found in equipment used in phlebotomy such as gloves, tourniquets, bandages, and tape. Health care workers and patients can be allergic to latex and can experience symptoms ranging from itchy, red, watery eyes to chest tightness, shortness of breath, or shock. Latex can also cause bumps, sores, or red raised areas on the part of the skin exposed to latex. Powdered gloves are especially dangerous because when the gloves are removed, the powder disperses into the air. If using latex gloves always wash your hands when removing the gloves and do not use oil-based creams or lotions that can cause the gloves to deteriorate. Powdered latex gloves should never be used for phlebotomy. Always ask the patient if he or she is allergic to latex if you are using any supplies or equipment that contain latex. If you or your patients have a latex allergy, all products containing latex *must* be avoided. In general, the smartest choice for the phlebotomist and patient is non-latex.

Patient Education & Communication

Gloves and Allergies

When describing the phlebotomy procedure to the patient, explain your legal requirement to wear gloves and be certain to ask the patient if he or she is allergic to latex. This will make the patient feel more comfortable and help prevent exposing a patient with allergies to latex products.

Alcohol Prep Pads

A venipuncture site must be cleaned prior to needle insertion. Infection at the site of needle insertion could occur if the area was not cleaned. **Antiseptic,** a germicidal solution, is used to clean the venipuncture site prior to needle insertion. One type of antiseptic frequently used, alcohol prep pads, are sterile pads saturated with 70% isopropyl alcohol. Seventy percent isopropyl alcohol is a **bacteriostatic** antiseptic, meaning that it inhibits the growth of bacteria. This prevents contamination by normal skin bacteria during a venipuncture. Alcohol preps are not recommended for the collection of blood alcohol levels or for dermal punctures when testing for blood glucose. Also, depending on the site or test, stronger antiseptics may be used. Collection of blood cultures or an arterial puncture require additional sterility; for these procedures antiseptics such as iodine or chlorhexidine gluconate are used to clean the puncture site.

Figure 3-6 A stretchy dressing such as **(a)** Coban® or a **(b)** roller gauze dressing is used to apply pressure to a venipuncture site and prevent exposing a patient to adhesive tape.

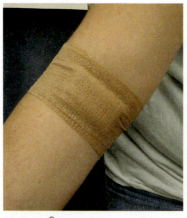

(a) Coban®

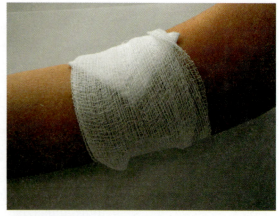

(b) Roller gauze

Gauze Pads

Gauze is a loosely woven cotton fabric that is applied with pressure to the arm immediately upon withdrawal of the needle following venipuncture. Along with applying pressure to the venipuncture site to ensure that bleeding has stopped, gauze can be folded into quarters and taped to the patient's skin to serve as a pressure bandage, which will maintain a firm amount of pressure to the site. In many cases a roller gauze is wrapped entirely around the arm so tape is not placed on the skin. A special Coban® bandage can also be used to apply pressure (see Figure 3-6).

Adhesive Bandage

An adhesive bandage, paper tape, or gauze is placed over the puncture site to stop the bleeding. When a patient has fragile skin, such as small children or the elderly, adhesive should not be placed directly on the skin. Latex-free tape and bandages should be used for patients with allergies. A patient should be advised to hold the arm straight, apply pressure for 3 to 5 minutes, and remove the bandage in 15 to 20 minutes. Avoiding lifing and frequent bending of the elbow are also important to prevent the return of bleeding.

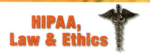

HIPAA, Law & Ethics

Remove the Tourniquet

Failure to remove the tourniquet following venipuncture can cause temporary or permanent injury to the patient. If the phlebotomist were to apply the tourniquet under the gown sleeve of an unconscious patient and forget to remove it after obtaining the blood specimen, tissues and cells in the affected limb would die. Prolonged blockage of blood to the affected limb could result in amputation because of this act of negligence.

Needles

The needle is composed of the hub, or plastic section; the shaft; and the **bevel,** or slanted tip at the point. **Sterile** needles (those free of microorganisms) are available in peel-apart packages or plastic cases. The tops or ends of needles

Figure 3-7 Needles are usually color-coded to indicate the size and/or gauge.

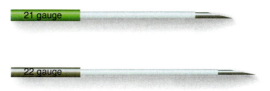

are usually color-coded to quickly identify the proper length and gauge of the needle, as a safety precaution (see Figure 3-7). The tip of the needle should be checked for damage or for burrs, which are small imperfections or rough edges on the end of the needle. These burrs will cause unnecessary pain for the patient. A blunt or bent tip can be harmful to the patient and interfere with collecting a blood sample. If using only disposable needles, the likelihood of having a damaged needle is small; however, you may occasionally encounter a "bad" needle. If you find a needle that is damaged, discard the needle in the sharps container and get a new needle.

Because of the large number of documented needlestick injuries, the Needlestick Safety and Prevention Act was put into place in 2001. This act states that needles used in phlebotomy should have special safety features to protect the phlebotomist from accidental puncture with a contaminated needle. In most cases the user must actively engage the safety feature. These safety features should be activated as soon as the procedure is completed. In many cases the device is designed to be activated before the needle is removed from the patient. Keep your hands behind the exposed needle when activating the safety feature and watch for the sign, such as an audible click or color change, that indicates the feature is engaged. Table 3-1 on page 70 provides examples of safe needle devices for phlebotomy.

Safety and Infection Control

Preventing Needlestick Injuries

Safety devices for phlebotomy will only prevent injury when activated correctly. Make sure you know how to activate the device you are using for phlebotomy. Failure to activate a safety device greatly increases your risk for a needlestick injury.

Patient Education & Communication

Preventing Allergies and Bleeding

Patients could be allergic to bandages or the adhesive used on the bandages. If your patient is allergic, bandages should not be used. Coban® or gauze wrapped completely around the arm can be used. If no bandage or dressing is applied, the patient should maintain pressure until bleeding has completely stopped, which usually takes 15 minutes. The patient should also be instructed not to lift anything or bend his or her arm too much to reduce the risk of dislodging the platelet plug. This could cause further bleeding or a hematoma.

TABLE 3-1 Safe-Needle Devices

Feature	Example	Activation
Self-blunting needle	Blood collection tube / Blunt-tip blood-drawing needle / Sharp point / Blunt point	After the blood is drawn, a push on the collection tube moves the blunt needle forward through the outer shell and past the needle point. The blunt point can be activated before it is removed from the vein or artery.
Self-blunting butterfly needle		After collection and before the removal of the needle, the wing is flipped to the other side, blunting the needle.
Hinged cap		Using the thumb, a protective hinged cap is flipped over the needle and locks into place.
Protective shield		The user slides a plastic cover over the needle and locks it in place. Syringes also have this device.
Retractable needle		The needle is spring-loaded and retracts into the barrel when a button is pushed to activate.

Needles vary in length from ¾ to 1½ inches. The bore size, or **gauge,** of the needle also varies from large, 16-gauge needles used to collect units of blood to smaller, 23-gauge needles used for very small veins. The smaller the number assigned to the gauge, the larger the bore size, or inside diameter, of the needle. The most commonly used sizes for venipuncture are 21 to 22 gauge and 1¼ to 1½ inches. A smaller gauge needle increases the risk of hemolysis. A needle over 1 inch provides greater control and ease of thumb placement during venipuncture. Butterfly needles are typically ¾ inch long.

A phlebotomist generally uses three types of needles: (1) a multiple-sample needle, used as part of an evacuated collection system (a double-pointed needle and collection tube that contains a vacuum); (2) a hypodermic needle, used with a **syringe;** and (3) a butterfly (wing-tipped) needle. The double-pointed needle has a rubber sleeve over one end of the needle and is designed so that one end is for the venipuncture and the other end is used to puncture the rubber stopper of the evacuated collection tube. This rubber sleeve makes it easier to draw multiple tubes because the sleeve covers the needle inside the tube holder (adapter), preventing blood from dripping into the holder before another tube is attached.

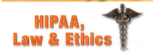

Reporting Needlestick Injuries

Whether you sustain a needlestick injury yourself or witness a co-worker being stuck, you must report the injury to your supervisor. In addition, you are obligated to report hazards from needles you observe in the workplace.

Evacuated Tube Holder

An **evacuated tube holder,** called a barrel or an adapter, is a specialized plastic adapter that holds both a needle and a tube for blood collection (see Figure 3-8). Needles are designed so that they can be screwed into a tube adapter that holds the evacuated tube. The evacuated tube holder has a flange at the end where the tube is inserted. This flange area is helpful during the venipuncture procedure. An evacuated tube holder is usually made of a clear, rigid plastic. These holders are to be discarded after use. Safety needles have an evacuated tube holder permanently attached to the needle. This whole assembly is disposed of in one piece as a safety measure. The holders come in two sizes, one for the usual adult-size collection tube and a smaller version for a pediatric-size tube (see Figure 3-9).

Sharps Container

Needle disposal containers, also known as "sharps containers," are designed to protect health care personnel from accidental needlesticks from a contaminated needle (see Figure 3-10). These containers come in a variety of shapes and sizes. Used needles, lancets, and other sharp items must be disposed of immediately in these special containers. To prevent possible

Figure 3-8 Various types of tube holders are used in phlebotomy.

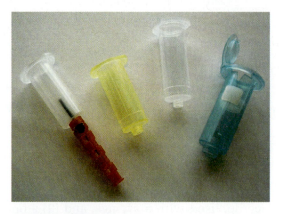

(a) Evacuated tube holders

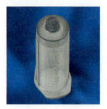

(b) Vacutainer® holder

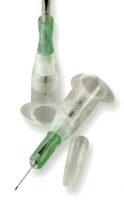

(c) BD Vacutainer®

needlesticks, the needle should not be removed from the holder manually. In this case the needle holder is disposed of in the sharps container as well. For protection and easy identification, sharps containers are made of non-penetrable material such as plastic and are red or bright orange, indicating a biohazard. Never open or tamper with a needle disposal container. These disposal units are marked with a biohazard label and are to be disposed of following biohazard guidelines established by OSHA.

Computer Label, Permanent Marker, or Pen

Each evacuated tube must be labeled at the time of specimen collection. Tubes must be labeled before the phlebotomist leaves the patient's side but never before the specimen is drawn. Tubes may be labeled with a computer-generated label or with a permanent marker or pen. Place the computer-generated label over the original tube label and not over the clear area of the tube. This will allow the amount and condition of the blood to be viewed during testing. When a computer label is used the phlebotomist must initial the tube after collection (see Figure 3-11). If computer labels are not provided, patient information must be written on the specimen labels of all tubes collected. Include the patient's name and identification number, the date and time of collection, and your initials. Specimens for the blood bank (such as type and cross-match) may have other special requirements such as bar-code identification.

Evacuated Tubes

Evacuated collection tubes contain a premeasured vacuum and are the most widely used system for blood collecting. Tubes come in a variety of sizes and colors. Sizes range from 2 to 15 milliliters. The colors vary based upon

Figure 3-9 Evacuated tubes range in size from 2 mL to 15 mL, and evacuated tube holders come in two sizes—adult and pediatric.

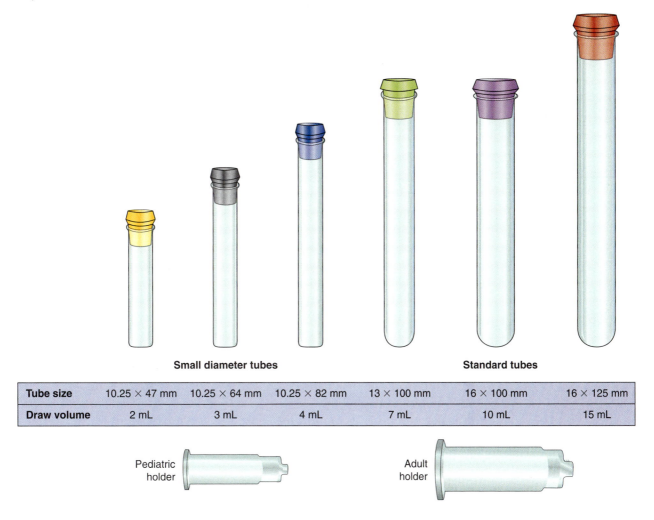

	Small diameter tubes				Standard tubes	
Tube size	10.25 × 47 mm	10.25 × 64 mm	10.25 × 82 mm	13 × 100 mm	16 × 100 mm	16 × 125 mm
Draw volume	2 mL	3 mL	4 mL	7 mL	10 mL	15 mL

Pediatric holder

Adult holder

Figure 3-10 All biohazardous sharps containers are closed systems and should not be opened. They can be **(a)** table top or **(b)** wall-mounted.

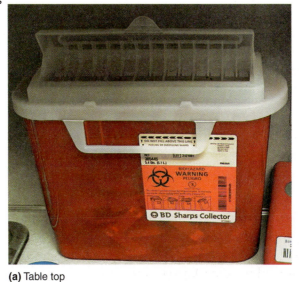

(a) Table top

(b) Wall-mounted

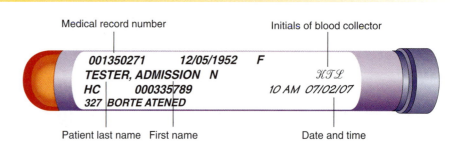

Figure 3-11 A computer label is used on the phlebotomy tube to ensure proper identification.

Medical record number

Initials of blood collector

001350271   12/05/1952   F
TESTER, ADMISSION   N
HC   000335789   *KTL*
327 BORTE ATENED   10 AM 07/02/07

Patient last name   First name

Date and time

the additives inside the tube and the type of test to be completed. Tubes are glass or plastic. Plastic tubes have less chance of breakage, thus preventing spillage and possible exposure to bloodborne pathogens. In the closed system of evacuated tubes, the patient's blood goes directly from the vein into a rubber-stoppered tube without being exposed to the air (see Figure 3-12). The evacuated tube system allows many tubes to be collected with one venipuncture. Evacuated tubes fill automatically with blood because a vacuum exists inside the tube. The vacuum inside the collection tube helps to "draw" the blood out of the patient's vein. The amount of vacuum is adequate for the tube to fill to the required amount for testing. Some evacuated collection tubes have a plastic splashguard that covers the sides of the tube. This splashguard is a safety device that helps reduce the **aerosol** mist (particles suspended in the air) that may be generated when the stopper of the tube is removed from the evacuated tube during specimen processing.

When multiple tubes are used for blood collection, the order in which you use the tubes is important. This is known as sequence, or "order of draw." For proper collection you should line up multiple evacuated tubes in the order of draw before starting the venipuncture. You should always double-check the requisition forms to make sure all appropriate tubes for tests ordered are available and ready before starting the venipuncture.

The most commonly used evacuated tubes and the **additive** in those tubes are shown in Table 3-2. Serum, the liquid portion of blood that has been allowed to clot, or coagulate, will form when blood is collected in a tube with no anticoagulant. Serum is blood without fibrinogen present because it is used up by making the clot. The clotted cells and serum will separate when centrifuged. Plasma is the result of blood collected in a tube that contains an anticoagulant. The anticoagulant in the evacuated tube prevents the specimen from clotting. This is the result of the anticoagulant neutralizing or removing one of the essential factors necessary for the clotting or coagulation process.

Figure 3-12 The evacuated collection tube assembly includes the **(a)** evacuated tube, **(b)** flange, **(c)** rubber stopper on the tube, **(d)** evacuated tube holder, and **(e)** needle (double-ended).

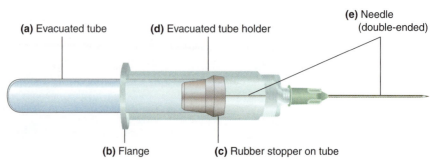

(a) Evacuated tube

(d) Evacuated tube holder

(e) Needle (double-ended)

(b) Flange

(c) Rubber stopper on tube

TABLE 3-2 Evacuated Tube Identification*

	Tube Color	Additive	Common Laboratory Use
	Red	None	Chemistry tests on serum: 　glucose 　cholesterol 　triglycerides 　HDL 　potassium 　amylase 　alkaline phosphatase 　BUN 　CK 　liver enzymes Serology tests on serum: 　RPR 　Monospot 　rheumatoid factor 　ANA
	Serum separator tube (SST)	Serum separator gel clot activator	Chemistry tests on serum: 　glucose 　cholesterol 　triglycerides 　potassium
	Lavender	EDTA	Hematology tests on whole blood: 　CBC 　differential 　platelet count 　reticulocyte count 　erythrocyte sedimentation rate 　sickle cell screen 　hemoglobin electrophoresis 　some chemistry tests 　hemoglobin A1c
	Light blue	Sodium citrate	Coagulation tests on plasma: 　PT 　APTT or PTT 　factor assays 　fibrinogen 　thrombin
	Green	Sodium heparin Lithium heparin Ammonium heparin	Chemistry tests on plasma: 　ammonia 　chromosome screening

	Tube Color	Additive	Common Laboratory Use
	Gray	Sodium fluoride Potassium oxalate	Glucose Lactate Alcohol levels
	Yellow	Sodium polyanethol sulfonate (SPS) Acid citrate dextrose (ACD)	Blood cultures Cellular studies HLA typing Paternity testing
	Light green or green/gray—Plasma separator tube (PST)	Lithium heparin and gel for plasma separation	Plasma tests in chemistry department STAT chemistry tests
	Orange or gray/yellow	Thrombin	STAT serum tests
	Royal blue	Clot activator (plastic serum) EDTA (plastic)	For trace elements, toxicology, and nutritional chemistry testing
	Tan	EDTA (plastic)	Lead
	White	EDTA with gel	Molecular diagnostic tests such as DNA testing
	Pink	Spray-coated EDTA	Whole blood hematology
	Clear or red/gray	None (plastic)	Used as a discard tube when required

*Adapted from BD Vacutainer® Tube Guide at www.bd.com/vacutainer.

It is important that tubes containing an anticoagulant be mixed or inverted gently several times (usually 8 to 10 times) immediately after drawing to ensure uniform mixing of the specimen with the anticoagulant. Check the manufacturer's directions for the proper number of inversions to perform.

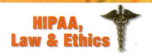

HIPAA, Law & Ethics

Follow Disposal Guidelines

All needles must be disposed of following biohazard guidelines. These guidelines are nationally mandated and locally regulated. If your used phlebotomy equipment ended up in the local landfill, you and your employer could face severe penalties.

Serum Separator Tubes

Serum separator tubes (SST) are used frequently in the chemistry section of the laboratory. Common tests performed in chemistry are glucose, cholesterol, triglycerides, and potassium. These tubes contain a clot activator and gel for serum separation.

Most SSTs have a speckled look, with black mixed into the red portion of the top. Some are gold topped. The clot activator speeds up the coagulation process, causing the sample to clot faster. The gel separates the serum from the blood cells by getting between the clot and the serum during centrifugation. Separating the serum from cells helps prevent contamination by cellular chemicals that are released because of hemolysis, which can occur within a couple of hours after collection. The gel separator makes it easier for laboratory personnel to obtain the serum for testing: with the gel in place the cells will not mix with the serum, making it easy to pour off the liquid for testing.

Red-Topped Tubes

Red-topped tubes come in glass or plastic. Glass tubes are recommended for serum testing. There is no additive or gel, thus making it easier to access the cells for testing.

Red-topped tubes are also used for most drug level tests. The drugs can sometimes get caught in the gel of an SST tube, lowering the results. Plastic red-topped tubes contain a clot activator and should not be used for blood banking.

Lavender-Topped Tubes

Lavender tubes are used frequently in the hematology section of the laboratory and in many blood banks. Common hematology tests performed are the CBC (complete blood cell count) and differential (percentage of each type of white cell). The additive in the lavender-topped tube is EDTA (ethylene-diamine-tetraacetic acid). EDTA prevents blood from clotting by binding with calcium. Since calcium is necessary for normal clot formation, when the EDTA binds with calcium, coagulation is prevented. EDTA is the anticoagulant of choice for hematology because it maintains the cells' shape and size better than other anticoagulants. EDTA also inhibits platelet clumping and does not interfere with routine staining procedures utilized in hematology.

Light Blue-Topped Tubes

Light blue-topped tubes are used in the coagulation section of the laboratory. Common coagulation tests performed are the prothrombin time (PT) and the activated partial thromboplastin time (APTT) or partial thromboplastin time (PTT). The primary additive or anticoagulant in the light blue-topped tube is sodium citrate. Like EDTA, sodium citrate binds calcium, thus preventing coagulation. In order to have accurate laboratory results this tube must be completely filled. Light blue-topped tubes have a relatively large amount of additive; therefore the ratio between blood collected and additive is more important than in other tubes with additives. Light blue-topped tubes also come in plastic.

In order to maintain the proper blood-to-additive ratio, the tube is completely filled during collection. The tube should be inverted to prevent clotting. When certain types of equipment are used for venipuncture, a small red tube may be collected first.

Green-Topped Tubes

Green-topped tubes contain the anticoagulant sodium heparin, lithium heparin, or ammonium heparin. Light green-topped or green-gray-topped tubes have lithium heparin and gel for plasma separation. These tubes are called plasma barrier tubes. PST™ is one brand of plasma barrier tube made by Becton Dickinson. Heparin stops the coagulation process by inactivating thrombin and thromboplastin, thus preventing clot formation. These tubes are used for tests requiring plasma. Many facilities use green-topped tubes for STAT and general chemistry tests.

Gray-Topped Tubes

Blood collected in gray-topped tubes is usually used for glucose analysis. Gray-topped tubes contain potassium oxalate (an anticoagulant), which stops the coagulation process by binding with calcium. All gray-topped tubes contain an **antiglycolytic** agent or glucose preservative such as sodium fluoride. A glycolytic inhibitor prevents the metabolism of glucose by red blood cells. These tubes are used for blood glucose and blood alcohol levels.

Yellow-Topped Tubes

Yellow-topped tubes are available with two different additives. The tubes look identical, but one contains sodium polyanethol sulfonate (SPS), which is used for blood culture collections. The other yellow-topped tube available contains acid citrate dextrose (ACD), which is an additive that maintains red cell viability and is used for cellular studies in blood banks or HLA typing. Discretion must be used when selecting a yellow-topped tube to ensure that the correct additive is present in the tube for the specific laboratory test ordered.

Troubleshooting

Hemolysis

You must select the appropriate tube size and needle for each blood collection. The phlebotomist must consider the amount of blood required and the size and condition of the patient's veins. If a small-bore needle is used with a large-volume tube, **hemolysis**—or destruction of red blood cells—of the sample collected can occur. Red blood cells are damaged when a large amount of vacuum causes them to be rapidly pulled through the small bore of a needle. Either a larger-bore needle should be used with a larger tube or a smaller tube should be used with a small-bore needle. Hemolysis of blood samples should be avoided at all costs. A hemolyzed sample will produce erroneous results for most laboratory tests.

Question: What should be done if a blood sample is hemolyzed?

_____

_____

_____

TABLE 3-3 Order of Draw for Multiple Tubes Using a Vacuum Tube System

1. Sterile specimens (blood culture tubes) or yellow SPS
2. Coagulation tubes (light blue-topped)*
3. SST (gold or red/black)
4. Serum (red plastic or glass)
5. Heparin (green)
6. PST (light-green or green/gray)
7. EDTA (pink or lavender)
8. Fluoride (glucose) (gray)

*When using a winged collection set, a discard tube is used to eliminate the dead air space and make certain the proper blood to additive ratio is maintained in the coagulation tube.

Order or Sequence of Draw

The order in which blood is collected using evacuated tube systems is critical for good test results. When collecting multiple specimens and specimens for coagulation tests, the order in which tubes are drawn can affect test results. Release of tissue thromboplastin from the skin as it is punctured can be present in the first tube collected. So if only a coagulation test (blue tube) is ordered, a small red/gray tube should be drawn first. This is essential if a butterfly assembly is used. The butterfly assembly is discussed later in this chapter. It is possible to contaminate tubes with anticoagulants from other tubes. This is why tubes that contain anticoagulants are drawn *after* the red-topped tubes. When sterile specimens are collected, such as with blood cultures (discussed in Chapter 5), they must be drawn first to prevent contamination from other tubes. Table 3-3 summarizes the order of draw for multiple tubes.

Butterfly Infusion Set with Syringe System

A **winged set** is commonly called a **butterfly needle set** because the plastic needle holder resembles butterfly wings; these attachments are used to hold the needle during insertion into the vein (see Figure 3-13). The butterfly set is not used as extensively as the evacuated blood collection system. With the higher cost and increased risk involved with butterfly or winged sets, many facilities recommend the use of a syringe with a small-gauge needle for smaller veins. You have just as much control, and can regulate the rate of blood extraction. One of the main reasons for butterfly sets is to have more control with non-stable patients. With nervous children, older patients with palsy, drunk or disorderly patients, or any instance where the patient may move or jerk during the draw, you can get the needle in, tape it down, and maintain stability for the entire draw and minimize the risk of vein damage due to excessive movement.

Older patients and children have small veins that may be too fragile to collect blood using the evacuated tube system. When the vacuum is applied, a fragile vein will tend to collapse, and the blood will not flow into the evacuated tube. The butterfly needle assembly is attached to flexible plastic tubing that can attach to a specially designed tube adapter or small syringe. This allows you to obtain the necessary amounts of blood while not

Figure 3-13 A butterfly or wing-tipped assembly is used for non-stable patients or in some cases of very small, fragile veins.

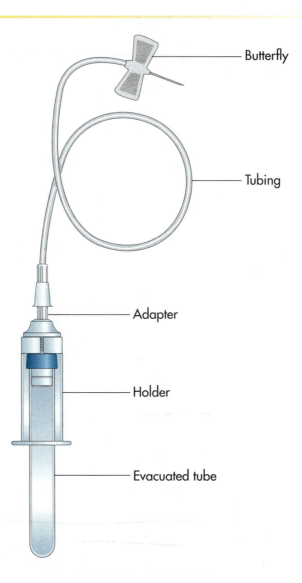

Butterfly

Tubing

Adapter

Holder

Evacuated tube

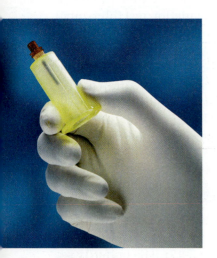

Figure 3-14 A syringe transfer device like this one should be used to prevent needlestick injuries when transferring blood from a syringe to a tube.

collapsing the vein with too much pressure or clotting the sample by having to go too slow with a large syringe. This system is completely sterile, and the syringe consists of a barrel and a plunger. The barrel usually is graduated in milliliters or fractions of a milliliter. The needle is fitted on the syringe by simply sliding the hub of the butterfly infusion set over the tip of the syringe. Butterfly infusion sets frequently have an adapter for the evacuated tube system. When a syringe is used, a transfer device must be used to avoid potential needlestick injury (see Figure 3-14).

✓ Checkpoint Questions 3-3

1. List all the equipment you will need to perform a venipuncture.

_____

_____

_____

_____

2. Why is it necessary to use different types of tubes for venipuncture?

_____

_____

_____

_____

3. If you were asked to perform a hemoglobin A1c and a cholesterol test, which tubes would you use in what order?

_____

_____

_____

_____

Answer the questions above and complete the *Specimen Collection Equipment* activity on the Student CD under Chapter 3 before you continue to the next section.

3-4 Dermal Puncture

Venipuncture is the most frequently performed phlebotomy procedure. However, because current laboratory instrumentation and procedures enable us to use smaller and smaller amounts of blood, obtaining microsamples by capillary or **dermal** (skin) puncture is also popular. Whenever a dermal puncture is performed it should be noted on the requisition slip. Microcollection, capillary puncture, and dermal puncture are generally used on infants and small children under two years of age. In some cases, microcollection by dermal puncture is performed on adult patients. Examples include cases of severe burns, situations in which veins are difficult to stick, patients who are receiving chemotherapy, older patients with very fragile veins, and patients performing home glucose monitoring for diabetes.

The blood collected by microcollection puncture comes from arterioles, venules, and capillaries and may contain small amounts of tissue fluid. Hemolysis is more frequently seen in specimens collected by dermal puncture. This is usually due to excessive squeezing of the puncture site in order to obtain enough specimen. Warming the site of dermal puncture increases bloodflow, thereby making the collection process much easier and reducing the amount of tissue fluid collected. For a dermal puncture sample, the concentration of glucose is slightly higher, whereas the concentrations of total protein, calcium, and potassium are slightly lower in blood obtained by dermal puncture versus venipuncture.

Dermal Puncture Collection Devices

Varieties of dermal puncture devices are available (see Figure 3-15). To prevent puncturing a bone, the puncture depth should not exceed 2.0 mm, especially when performing heel sticks on infants. Lancets are designed to control the depth of the dermal puncture. Safety lancets must be used, so

Figure 3-15 Dermal puncture devices must not puncture more than 2 mm into the skin and have retractable needles that retract after use.

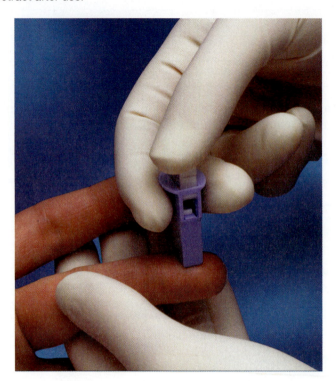

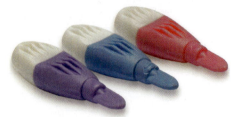

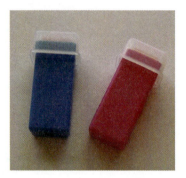

that the blade retracts after use to prevent needlestick injuries. To produce adequate bloodflow, the depth of the puncture is actually less important than the *width* of the incision. This is because the major vascular area of the skin is located near the surface of the skin, usually within 2 mm of the surface.

Most of the same equipment used for venipuncture is also used for dermal or capillary puncture. This equipment is usually assembled on a portable tray with handles or in a basket, for easy transport to the patient for blood collection. Required equipment for both procedures are gloves, alcohol pads, sterile gauze, and a sharps disposal container. In addition, some sort of microspecimen container is needed. Finally, because warming the site of puncture will increase bloodflow, a warm towel, cloth, or heel warmer packet should be available for a dermal puncture.

Varieties of microspecimen containers are available for collection of **microsamples** (samples of less than one milliliter). Some containers are designed for a specific test, whereas others are used for multiple purposes (see Figure 3-16). Some containers have a strawlike or scoop device to collect drops of blood. On the other hand, capillary tubes are used to collect the blood sample through the process of **capillary action.** Capillary action is the physical process of blood flowing, or being pulled, into a very thin tube. Capillary action eliminates the need to tip the tube downward, thus reducing the risk of getting air bubbles in the sample.

Capillary tubes or microhematocrit tubes are usually collected when a hematocrit is requested. A hematocrit is a blood test that is used to help detect anemia. Microhematocrit tubes are small plastic tubes or glass tubes with a thin Mylar filament wrapping. The use of a wrapped tube or

Figure 3-16 Microspecimen containers include small containers such as this Microtainer® by Becton Dickenson. Follow the manufacturer's instructions when filling any type of microspecimen container.

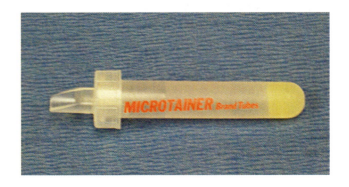

Figure 3-17 A capillary tube with clay sealant is used for microspecimens.

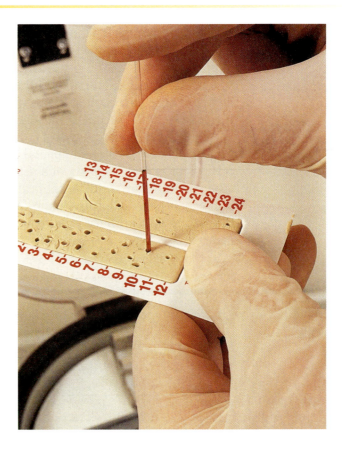

plastic tube has been adapted because of easy breakage of capillary tubes in the past. Three types of capillary tubes are available: red-tipped tubes, blue-tipped tubes, and black-tipped tubes. Red-tipped capillary tubes are coated on the inside with heparin (an anticoagulant) to prevent clotting of the specimen. Red-tipped capillary tubes are used to measure the hematocrit. When sufficient blood has been collected in the red-tipped capillary tube, one end of the capillary tube is closed by embedding it in a clay sealant designed for this use (see Figure 3-17). Also available are self-sealing capillary tubes that require no clay sealant after collection; however, care must be taken to collect from the opposite end of the sealant. Blue-tipped capillary tubes have no anticoagulant coating the inside, so specimens will clot in these tubes. Blue-tipped capillary tubes are used when no anticoagulant is required. Black-tipped tubes have a smaller diameter in order to collect a smaller amount of blood for centrifuged hematocrits.

Microcollection containers are usually plastic tubes that provide a larger collection volume than capillary tubes. Microtainers®, manufactured by Becton Dickinson, are one such type of collection device. Microcollection containers or devices come with a variety of anticoagulants, very much like the evacuated tube system, and use the same color-coded system. Some of these microcollection devices come with a scoop-collector top and others have a capillary type of device for collection. The scoop-type device is taken off after collection, and a color-coded cap is attached before mixing. Microcollection devices are mixed in the same way as evacuated tubes. Invert or mix the specimen eight to ten times by tilting or carefully inverting the capped device. It should be noted that proper mixing is just as important with the microcollection devices as with full-size evacuated tubes with anticoagulants. Without proper mixing of anticoagulant and specimen, the specimen will clot, and a clotted specimen *cannot* be used for laboratory testing. These microcollection tubes can be **centrifuged** in order to separate the cells from the serum or plasma.

For some hematology tests, diluted whole blood can be used. Becton Dickinson has developed special devices called Unopettes® for this purpose. The system consists of a sealed plastic reservoir containing a measured amount of fluid, a calibrated glass capillary pipette in a plastic holder, and a plastic pipette shield. The amount of diluent or fluid and the size of the capillary pipette are dependent on the laboratory test to be measured.

Checkpoint Questions 3-4

1. What type of patients typically require a dermal puncture?

_____

_____

_____

_____

2. Name and describe three types of microhematocrit tubes.

_____

_____

_____

_____

_____

Answer the questions above and complete the *Dermal Puncture* activity on the Student CD under Chapter 3 before you continue to the next section.

Chapter Summary

- The requisition will contain all or part of the following information depending upon your facility: name, date, time, ordering physician, type of test, medical record number, Social Security number, date of birth, test status, patient location, and initials of phlebotomist. All tube labels MUST include the patient's name, date, time, and the phlebotomist's initials.

- Computer information systems in phlebotomy are used to maintain patient data and results, receive orders, print requisitions, and generate patient charges.

- Equipment and supplies needed for phlebotomy include gloves; tourniquet; alcohol prep pads; gauze pads; adhesive bandage or tape; needles, evacuated tube holder, or syringe; sharps container; permanent marker, pen, or computer labels; and evacuated tubes.

- Evacuated tubes are a closed system of collection that allows for multiple tubes to be collected with one venipuncture.

- Used needles, sharps, and in many cases the tube holder must be disposed of in a sharps container made of nonpenetrable materials and bright red and orange biohazardous label.

- Evacuated tubes come in different colors with different additives and are designated for different tests based upon their additives. You should be familiar with the most common tube colors used at the facility where you are employed.

- The order of the draw is blood culture or yellow SPS tube, SST, serum tube—glass or plastic, heparin tubes (green), PST tube, EDTA tubes, pink or lavender, then gray tube.

- The winged-set includes a needle that has butterfly wings; short, thin tubing; and a place to attach a syringe or evacuated tube for blood collection. The syringe set, although used infrequently, includes a needle and syringe plus a transfer device for adding blood to the evacuated blood tubes.

- Dermal puncture is performed with a safety lancet or puncture device, special collection tubes, and the same equipment used for venipuncture.

Chapter Review

True or False

Place T or F in the space provided to indicate whether you think the statement is true or false. Correct the false statements to make them true.

_____ **1.** A requisition form requires a physician's signature.

_____ **2.** Non-latex gloves are the best choice for the phlebotomist and patient.

_____ **3.** Tourniquets cause the veins to enlarge or expand.

_____ **4.** A bacteriostatic antiseptic causes the skin to be contaminated with bacteria.

_____ **5.** The three parts to a needle are the hub, bevel, and shaft.

_____ **6.** Yellow-topped tubes are available with two different additives. One contains sodium polyanethol sulfonate and the other one contains sodium heparin.

_____ **7.** Sharps containers are bright orange and soft plastic or metal.

_____ **8.** The powder inside latex gloves can cause latex allergies.

Labeling

Label the numbered parts in the diagram with the correct name for each part.

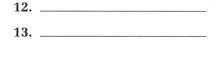

9. _____

10. _____

11. _____

12. _____

13. _____

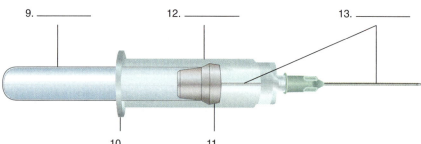

Matching

Match each definition with the correct term. Place the appropriate letter on the line to the left of each definition.

_____ **14.** anticoagulant

_____ **15.** gauge

_____ **16.** winged infusion set

_____ **17.** evacuated tube

_____ **18.** 23

a. Smallest needle gauge routinely used for blood collection.

b. Specialized plastic holder containing both the needle and the blood collection tube.

c. Closed collection tube containing a premeasured vacuum.

d. Strong antiseptic used when patients are allergic to iodine.

e. Also known as a butterfly needle.

_____ **19.** evacuated tube holder

_____ **20.** chlorhexidine gluconate

f. Agent that prevents blood from clotting.

g. Refers to the needle diameter or bore.

Fill in the Blanks

Next to each additive listed, write the color of the tube containing that additive.

Additive or Use	Tube Color or Type
21. sodium citrate	_____
22. none	_____
23. EDTA	_____
24. sodium fluoride/potassium oxalate	_____
25. sodium heparin/lithium heparin/ammonium heparin	_____

Ordering

For the following types of specimens to be drawn, indicate the correct order of draw (1 = first; 2 = second; and so on).

26. Light blue (coagulation) _____

27. Sterile specimens (blood cultures or yellow SPS tube) _____

28. Pink or lavender (EDTA) _____

29. Light green or green/gray (PST) _____

30. Gold or red/black (SST) _____

31. Red plastic or glass (serum) _____

32. Green (heparin) _____

33. Gray (fluoride) _____

Multiple Choice

Circle the correct answer.

34. The term "evacuated tube" refers to a venipuncture collection tube that:
    a. Does not contain a vacuum
    b. Contains a vacuum
    c. Does not contain an anticoagulant
    d. Contains an anticoagulant

35. The purpose of an anticoagulant in a blood collection tube is to:
    a. Decrease the chance of hemolysis
    b. Preserve the life span of red blood cells
    c. Prevent blood from clotting
    d. Produce serum for testing

36. When performing a venipuncture on a patient with small veins, the best size of needle to use is:
   a. 16 gauge
   b. 18 gauge
   c. 20 gauge
   d. 22 gauge

37. Gloves are required for:
   a. Transporting specimens to the lab
   b. A new phlebotomist performing a venipuncture
   c. An experienced phlebotomist performing a venipuncture
   d. All of the above

38. It is necessary to control the depth of a dermal puncture device during capillary collection in order to:
   a. Puncture an artery
   b. Control excessive clotting
   c. Avoid puncturing a bone
   d. Avoid bacterial contamination

39. A _____ is a blood test that is used to help detect anemia.
   a. hematocrit
   c. dermal puncture
   b. chemistry panel
   d. none of the above

40. To prevent puncturing a bone, the puncture depth should not exceed _____, especially when performing heel sticks on infants.
   a. 2.4 mm
   b. 2.0 mm
   c. 2.8 mm
   d. None of the above

41. The correct sequence or order of draw is as follows:
   a. Green, lavender, gray
   b. Gray, lavender, green
   c. Lavender, gray, green
   d. None of the above

42. There are at least four major items needed when correctly filling out the label on a tube of blood:
   a. Patient's name, date, time, phlebotomist initials
   b. Patient's name, date, time, and test to be performed
   c. Name, date, test to be performed, physician's name
   d. None of the above

What Should You Do?

In the space provided, describe what you would do in the following situations. Use critical thinking and troubleshooting. Be sure to include the reason for your decision.

43. You are a phlebotomist preparing to collect a blood specimen from a patient. When you open the sealed package containing the needle, you find the needle to be slightly bent. What would you do and why?

_____

_____

44. Blood has been ordered drawn from a 4-month-old child. You must decide on the best equipment to use in this instance. What would you use and why?

_____

_____

45. As a phlebotomist you are trained to wear gloves during every procedure. What would you do if you suspect you are allergic to latex? What would you do if your patient is allergic to latex?

_____

_____

_____

46. You have been asked to draw the following blood tests. For each patient determine what tubes you will use in what order?

    a. Patient #1 Ordered: CBC, PT, and PTT

_____

_____

    b. Patient #2 Ordered: Cholesterol, triglycerides

_____

_____

    c. Patient #3 Ordered: Blood culture, potassium, and alcohol level

_____

_____

Get Connected _Internet Activity_

Visit the McGraw-Hill Higher Education Online Learning Center _Phlebotomy for Health Care Personnel_ Website at **www.mhhe.com/healthcareskills** to complete the following activities.

    1. Safe-needle devices must be used in phlebotomy to prevent accidental needlesticks. Go to the Occupational Safety and Health Administration Website and review the latest requirements for safe-needle devices. Write a brief summary of the guidelines for all safe-needle devices.

    2. Visit the Websites of phlebotomy equipment manufacturers to become familiar with the various evacuated tubes (Vacutainers®) used in phlebotomy. Develop a poster, chart, or presentation to help you identify and remember the colors, additives, tests completed, and proper order of the draw.

 # Using the Student CD

Now that you have completed the material in the chapter text, return to the Student CD and complete any chapter activities you have not yet done. Practice your terminology with the "Key Term Concentration" game. Review the chapter material with the "Spin the Wheel" game. Take the final chapter test and complete the troubleshooting question and e-mail or print your results to document your proficiency for this chapter.

4 Performing Venipuncture and Dermal Puncture

Chapter Outline

Learning Outcomes

Upon completion of this chapter, you should be able to:

- Describe the proper procedure to follow for patient identification.
- Explain how to prepare a patient for blood collection.
- Identify the correct steps to follow when a patient refuses collection.
- Describe the process and time limits for applying a tourniquet to a patient's arm.
- Discuss factors that must be considered when selecting a site for venipuncture or dermal puncture.
- Describe the venipuncture and dermal puncture site cleansing procedure.
- List the items required on a specimen label and explain the importance of each.
- State the maximum number of times that the phlebotomist should stick a patient.
- List the steps to follow when unable to obtain a blood specimen.
- Describe how to use a butterfly or wing-tipped collection device.
- Explain the collection procedure for dermal puncture.

Key Terms

basal state	fasting
bedside manner	hemoconcentration
calcaneus	interstitial fluid
collapsed vein	lymphostasis
concentric circles	osteomyelitis
ecchymosis	palmar
edema	palpate
edematous	peak level

petechiae
plantar
postprandial
sclerosis

supine
syncope
trough level
venous reflux

4-1 Introduction

The routine venipuncture and dermal puncture procedures include a series of detailed steps that must be performed safely and accurately. Following aseptic technique and standard precautions and obtaining the specimen in the correct container are essential. Accurate patient identification and proper preparation are mandatory. To be a phlebotomist you must be able to perform venipuncture and dermal puncture proficiently.

Checkpoint Question 4-1

1. What are essential elements of the venipuncture and dermal puncture procedure?

_____

_____

_____

_____

4-2 Preparing for Venipuncture

The phlebotomist must have a certain level of confidence before meeting the patient. Knowing how to perform the proper technique may not be sufficient, because the patient's veins may not be a textbook example. Sometimes there may be a reason a particular arm may not be used. The patient may be scared, anxious, or combative in nature. In such instances, self-confidence combined with experience provides the mind-set required to successfully obtain the specimen on even the most difficult draws.

Greeting the Patient

The phlebotomist sets the tone for the venipuncture procedure when he or she greets the patient (see Figure 4-1). Smile and address the patient in a calm, pleasant tone of voice to gain the patient's confidence and trust. Behave as a professional. A professional manner includes behavior, appearance, courtesy, and respect toward the patient. Treat each patient the way you would want to be treated. This is called **bedside manner.** A confident manner will put the patient at ease as well as divert the patient's attention from the phlebotomy procedure. When greeting a patient you should always identify yourself. In most cases it would be appropriate to state your first name. However keeping your last name private is the better choice in some circumstances. A patient may become upset about treatment or become affectionate to you and attempt to contact you outside of the facility. For these reasons, many facilities recommend you simply identify yourself as from the

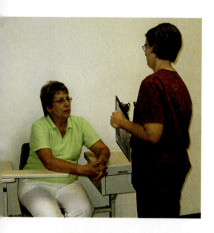

Figure 4-1 Greet the patient with a smile and use a calm tone to gain the patient's confidence and trust.

lab, or by using your first name only. Check the policy of the facility where you are employed. In either case, after identifying yourself, be certain to state why you are there and what you will be doing. Remember, you represent the laboratory profession.

Greeting the patient properly is important for both inpatients and outpatients. Outpatient situations include areas designated in a hospital or clinic, a patient's home, long-term health care facilities, and physician offices, among others, as discussed in Chapter 2. In an outpatient situation, the first few seconds are even more critical than with an inpatient. If a patient is in a hospital, it is not a surprise for a phlebotomist to arrive to collect a specimen, but in an outpatient situation, your arrival may not be expected. When a patient is not in a traditional hospital or clinic setting, a person arriving to collect a blood sample would not be a usual visitor; therefore, your arrival may cause the patient to become anxious. Conducting yourself in a professional manner is essential for these outpatient situations.

Inpatients present different situations. Doors to most patients' rooms are usually open. Whether a patient's door is closed or open, knock and wait for a response before entering. In some cases a patient cannot respond, especially if he is asleep or has been sedated or has a medical appliance covering or inserted into the mouth. After knocking, wait a few seconds for a response before entering the room. Open the door slowly, and greet the patient before proceeding into the room. Even if the door is slightly ajar, it is still a good idea to knock lightly to make the patient aware that you are about to enter. Sometimes the curtain is pulled around the patient's bed. Treat this situation in a similar manner. Talk to the patient through the curtain before pulling it back and entering. Taking this small extra step before entering the patient's room could save you and the patient embarrassment in the event the patient is undergoing a procedure or using a bedpan or urinal. Following these steps will make the patient feel respected and help create a positive attitude for the phlebotomy procedure.

Patient Education & Communication

Difficult Patients

Patients often do not feel well. They may be angry or scared about their medical condition. The patient could take out his frustration or anger on the phlebotomist. Regardless of what the patient says or how the patient acts, the phlebotomist must remain polite and professional. Whatever happens or is said to you, do not take it personally. Being polite and as kind as possible is the easiest way to improve an unpleasant situation.

Troubleshooting

Wake the Patient Gently

During early morning blood collections the patient may be asleep. Gently wake him or her and explain why you are there. Try not to startle the patient. Nudge the bed, instead of touching the patient. Talk in a soft manner and avoid turning on bright lights. Inform the patient before turning on a light to give him or her the opportunity to shield the eyes. Never attempt to collect a specimen from a sleeping patient—you could injure yourself or the patient if he or she were to startle awake and jerk the arm.

Question: How can you avoid startling the patient who is sleeping?

_____

_____

_____

If the patient is not in the room, proceed to the nurses' station to check where the patient is and when the patient is expected back. This is especially important if the specimen to be collected is a STAT (immediately) or timed specimen, which will be discussed in Chapter 6. Make every attempt to locate the patient, because sometimes the patient is only walking in the hallway or could be undergoing a procedure in another part of the hospital. If you cannot locate the patient or the patient has not returned within a reasonable length of time, inform the appropriate person (nurse or ward clerk) at the nurses' station that the specimen was not collected. Document on the request slip the time and name of the person you spoke with at the nurses' station. Ask that the laboratory be informed when the patient returns. Inform the laboratory supervisor that the patient specimen was not collected in case the laboratory is called for results later.

Patient Identification

The most important step in the venipuncture procedure is proper identification of the patient. It makes no difference how sophisticated or expensive the laboratory equipment is on which the specimen is tested; the results will be wrong if collected from the wrong patient. If this occurs, the results could be disastrous. Phlebotomists have been fired due to lack of proper patient identification. Say, for instance, that a blood specimen was collected for a cross-match because Mr. W. Buller is having surgery. But the cross-match specimen was collected from a Mr. B. Buller instead. After Mr. W. Buller's surgery he was given the unit of blood the doctor had requested. However, it was an incorrect cross-match, resulting in the wrong blood being administered. Mr. W. Buller could suffer serious consequences ranging from minor transfusion reactions to death if this error were to occur.

A potentially serious consequence of inaccurate patient identification could also occur when drug or medication levels are drawn. A physician needs to know if the dose of a medication is at the appropriate amount or level. A drug peak level may be requested. A **peak level** is a specimen collected when the serum drug level is at its highest level, shortly after a medication is given. The laboratory results for the peak level determine the amount of medicine the physician orders for the patient's next dose. If the wrong patient was drawn and the wrong peak level given to the physician, who then prescribed the wrong dose, the patient could become ill or even die. While these are extreme cases, these unfortunate patient identification errors have occurred and could still happen. The most important step in a venipuncture procedure is proper patient identification.

Always ask the patient to state his or her name and date of birth. Never ask, "Are you Mr. Ward?" A person who is on medication or is a heavy sleeper may answer "Yes" to any question you ask. Allow the patient to answer fully, not just say yes or no. Ask for the information you have on the requisition form. You could also ask the patient for his or her address if this is supplied on the form. Remember, you must verify at least two patient identifiers before proceeding. You can also double-check information provided to you visually. For example, does the patient match the age and sex given on the requisition form? These suggestions will help ensure that the proper patient's specimen is collected.

Identification of Inpatients

For inpatients always look at the identification (ID) band on the arm of the patient (see Figure 4-2). Does the identification number on the armband match the one on the requisition form? Does the information on the ID band exactly match the information on the requisition? You must use at least two identifiers, such as name, birth date, and/or medical record number. Both identifiers must match the requisition. *Even if there is only one number or letter difference, you cannot proceed with the venipuncture.* Never rely on the information on a card or ID band that is taped to the door, wall, or end of the bed. Patients are often transferred from room to room or out of the hospital without this information being changed. The only dependable information is on the patient's wristband. Unfortunately, patients could exchange wristbands. Though this occurrence is rare, it is best both to check the wristband and to ask the patient questions. If there is a discrepancy, ask for assistance from the patient's nurse.

Figure 4-2 Check the identification bracelet of an inpatient. In some cases, you will scan the bracelet for proper identification.

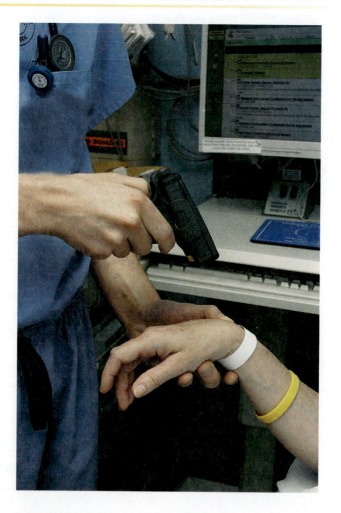

In some circumstances the ID band may not be present on the patient's wrist. If this should occur, look to see if the ID band was placed on the ankle instead. An ID band may be placed on the ankle because of burns, amputation, or **edema** (swelling) of the arm. If no ID band is found, do not perform the venipuncture until the ID band is located and properly attached to the patient's arm and the identification of the patient has been verified.

If the patient is unable to speak due to being sedated, in a coma, or on a ventilator, the patient's nurse will need to come to the patient's room to give verbal verification of the patient's identity. The phlebotomist should compare verbal information with the patient's armband and the requisition. Sometimes you will be expected to collect a specimen from an unconscious or nonresponsive patient. You must still identify yourself and inform the patient of the procedure you are about to perform. Unconscious patients may still be able to hear what is being said to them; they just cannot respond. An unconscious patient may be able to feel pain, so you should be prepared for the patient to move once you have inserted the needle. You may need to have someone assist you in holding the arm steady. Since the patient will not be able to apply adequate pressure after the venipuncture, the phlebotomist must apply pressure until the site has stopped bleeding.

Patient Education & Communication

Explain the Procedure

As a part of informed consent, it is the phlebotomist's responsibility to inform the patient of the pending procedure. The phlebotomist must briefly describe the venipuncture procedure. The phlebotomist must determine that the patient understands what is about to take place. Most people have had a blood test before; therefore the explanation "I'm here to draw your blood" should be sufficient. However, the patient may not understand English; in that case the phlebotomist must use sign language, a demonstration of a venipuncture, or some other means to get the idea of the venipuncture procedure across to the patient. Explaining the procedure to a family member who speaks English may be helpful if the family member is then able to provide the explanation to the patient. If this fails, you must locate an interpreter before the procedure can continue.

Identification of Outpatients

An outpatient normally does not have an armband or identification band. The same is usually true of patients in an emergency department. Outpatients usually arrive in the laboratory area with a physician order form or prescription form listing the requested laboratory tests. After the receptionist has filled out the laboratory requisition forms, the phlebotomist must verify the patient's identification by asking for some sort of identification card and requesting the patient state his or her full name and date of birth. The phlebotomist must ask the patient to verify the information on the lab requisition form. Information to verify includes date of birth, physician's name, ID number (if it appears on the laboratory requisition form), and maybe even the patient's home address or telephone number. This does not have to be a prolonged identification; usually two or three verification items are sufficient to ensure proper identification. In the emergency room when a patient without an identification band cannot respond, you must ensure correct identification through the licensed practitioner at the bedside.

Verifying Dietary Restrictions

After properly identifying the patient and obtaining patient consent to the phlebotomy procedure, you must verify any special dietary restrictions or instructions. Laboratory tests can be affected by what a patient eats or doesn't eat, or even by whether the patient has smoked within a designated time. To verify that a patient has followed instructions (given when the test was ordered), simply ask, "When was the last time you had anything to eat, drink, or smoke?" The most common dietary restriction that affects specimen collection is called **fasting,** which means the specimen needs to be drawn after the patient has not ingested foods or liquids for a specified period of time. Routinely the fast is for 12 hours, but in some instances a fast of 4, 8, or 16 hours may be requested by the licensed practitioner. When the patient has fasted for 12 hours and has not exercised, this is referred to as a **basal state.** This is the metabolic condition of the body usually during early morning collections. Some laboratory tests require special diet instructions. The patient may be instructed to eat or not eat certain foods for a specified number of days or hours before the specimen is taken. A common test request is for a 2-hour **postprandial** glucose test. This laboratory specimen must be drawn two hours after the patient has eaten, usually after breakfast. If a restriction or special diet is required and the patient followed this requirement, make a notation of this on the requisition slip. Make a note on the requisition of the last time the patient said he had anything to eat, drink, or smoke, and note if special dietary instructions were followed or not.

Patient Education & Communication

Dietary Restrictions Not Followed

Sometimes a patient forgets or is not informed of the dietary restrictions necessary before blood is drawn. In these circumstances you will need to ask the licensed practitioner if a nonfasting specimen will be adequate. In some instances this will be allowed. A few laboratory tests have little difference in normal value if the patient was nonfasting before the specimen was drawn. However, for some tests, especially glucose and lipid profiles, the specimen has to be fasting. If the licensed practitioner approves collecting the nonfasting specimen, note "nonfasting" on both the tube and laboratory requisition. Additionally, make a notation on the laboratory requisition of the person who approved taking the nonfasting specimen. It is good practice to notify the laboratory section performing the test that the licensed practitioner approved the nonfasting sample. Some laboratories will not report results if proper patient procedures (such as fasting) were not followed unless approval is noted.

Figure 4-3 Assemble the equipment for venipuncture.

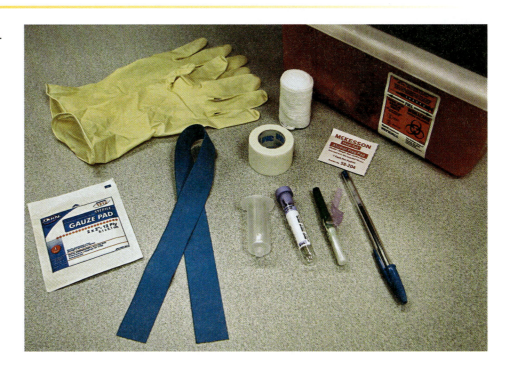

Assembling the Venipuncture Equipment

Collect and assemble all supplies needed for the venipuncture (see Figure 4-3). As you will recall from Chapter 3, a routine venipuncture uses the following items:

- Gloves
- Tourniquet
- Alcohol prep pads
- Gauze pads
- Needle
- Evacuated tube holder or syringe
- Appropriate evacuated tubes
- Needle disposal (sharps) container
- Adhesive bandage or tape
- Permanent marker, pen, or computer labels

Line up the venipuncture equipment near the patient. Attach the needle into the tube adapter and verify that the needle–tube adapter assembly is secure. Venipuncture equipment is made by many manufacturers, so make sure the tube adapter and needle are made by the same company or manufacturer. The adapters and needles are not interchangeable. Make sure that the needle is screwed all the way up to the tube adapter. Insert the first tube to be collected into the tube adapter. Push up to the adapter guideline or indentation in the tube adapter, or simply stabilize the tube with your small finger as you prepare to insert the needle. Check the directions of the equipment you are using and your facility's guidelines. In either case, be especially careful not to push the tube too hard because this would result in a loss of vacuum in the tube (see Figure 4-4).

Figure 4-4 Complete venipuncture assembly.

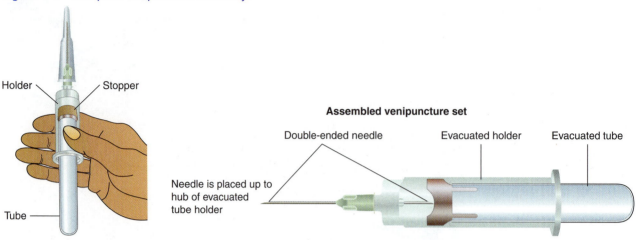

Troubleshooting **Patient Refusal**

Sometimes a patient will refuse to have his or her blood drawn. Explain that the physician ordered the test and the test results are needed to help diagnose or treat their medical condition. If the patient still refuses, do not attempt to draw blood. It is the patient's right to refuse the procedure, and the phlebotomist should not badger or restrain the patient in order to perform the procedure. Inform the licensed practitioner of the patient's refusal and note on the laboratory requisition that the patient refused the procedure. Be sure to document on the requisition the name of the licensed practitioner that you informed about this, along with the date, time, and your initials. You should also inform the phlebotomy supervisor of the situation.

Question: What should be written on the requisition when a patient refuses venipuncture?

_____

_____

_____

Patient Positioning

The position of the patient is another critical factor for a successful venipuncture. The patient should be either lying down or sitting in a special phlebotomy chair designed for outpatients. Most phlebotomy chairs have a movable arm support that helps in positioning the patient's arm (see Figure 4-5). Never attempt a phlebotomy procedure with a patient standing. It is uncomfortable for the patient, and if the patient were to get dizzy or faint, he or she could fall and be injured. A stool is not acceptable either because it is too unstable. Not all phlebotomy locations have the specially designed phlebotomy chair.

If a phlebotomy chair is not available, a phlebotomy procedure can still be performed. A straight chair with an arm is preferable to a chair without arms. The arm of the chair will aid in the support of the patient's

Figure 4-5 The arm supports on this outpatient phlebotomy chair are designed for comfort and correct positioning of the patient during outpatient phlebotomy procedures.

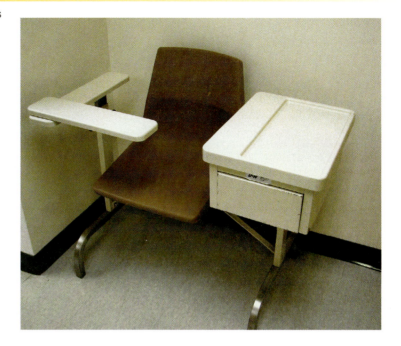

arm during the procedure. If only an armless chair is available, the patient will need to place the arm on the thigh for proper support during the phlebotomy. If an armless chair is used, the phlebotomist should position the chair against a wall or some other stable object. If the patient were to faint, the phlebotomist could then push the patient against the wall to keep him or her from falling out of the chair. If necessary, a pillow or rolled up towel placed under the patient's arm can be used to position the arm. When the patient is seated the arm needs to be supported and should extend downward in a straight line from the shoulder to the wrist. The arm should not be bent at the elbow.

Inpatients usually are in their hospital beds for the phlebotomy procedure. Therefore the **supine** position, with the patient lying on the back, face upward, is the most common phlebotomy position. The arm should be extended in a straight line from the shoulder and not bent. A rolled towel or pillow can be used to support the arm and aid in positioning the arm in a downward fashion. Hyperextending the elbow slightly can help the phlebotomist locate a vein. Bedrails are a major concern when performing venipuncture in a hospital situation. If you lower the bedrail for a procedure, you must raise it back before leaving the room.

Applying the Tourniquet

The placement of a tourniquet on the arm makes the veins more visible and will help you decide which vein to use. When a tourniquet is applied, the flow of venous blood is slowed, which increases pressure in the veins, making them more visible and palpable (or noticeable by touch). Application of a tourniquet makes it easier to feel, or **palpate,** the vein for possible venipuncture. A tourniquet is applied three to four inches above the venipuncture site, which is usually inside the elbow so the tourniquet is placed above the elbow. The tourniquet should not pinch the patient's skin, but it should feel slightly tight. However, it should not be so tight

Figure 4-6 Tourniquet on arm.

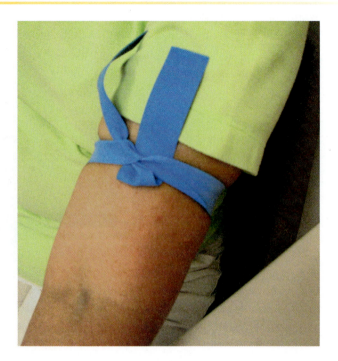

that the arm goes numb or turns colors. For the added comfort of the patient, you should avoid twisting the tourniquet. A twisted tourniquet will pinch and feel as if it is digging into the patient's arm, causing unnecessary discomfort and pain. The tourniquet should be kept flat against the arm in order to avoid this discomfort to the patient (see Figure 4-6). If a patient has fragile skin, you should try to place the tourniquet over his or her sleeve. If the patient is wearing a shirt without sleeves, place a hand towel or washcloth over the skin, then place the tourniquet over the towel to reduce the risk of tearing the skin or creating any damage to the patient's arm.

Position the tourniquet under the arm while grasping the ends above the arm and venipuncture area. Cross the left end over the right end, and apply a small amount of tension to the tourniquet. Grasp both ends of the tourniquet close to the patient's arm between the thumb and forefinger of the left hand. Using the right middle finger or index finger, tuck the left end under the right end. The loose end of the tourniquet will be pointing toward the shoulder and the loop will be pointed toward the hand (see Figure 4-7). When tugged after the venipuncture procedure, the loose end will easily release the tourniquet from the arm.

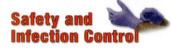

Safety and Infection Control

Areas Not Designed for Blood Collection

In most cases you will be drawing blood in outpatient and inpatient facilities that are designed for blood collection and the necessary materials will be at hand. However, you may become employed as a phlebotomist in the community at a location not typically used for blood collection. Organization in this type of environment is key to safety. Consider using the 1-2-3-2-1 method to ensure you are set for the procedure.

1—pair of gloves

2—tourniquet and alcohol swab

3—needle, sleeve, and tubes (in the order to be drawn)

2—gauze/cotton swab and bandage

1—sharps container

Making sure you have each of these pieces of equipment in this order will ensure you are prepared. Also be certain to have available and close by additional tubes and needles in case they are needed.

Troubleshooting **Petechiae**

Petechiae, or small, nonraised red spots on the skin due to a minute hemorrhage, can result if a tourniquet is left on too long. Petechiae may be seen in normal patients and patients with coagulation disorders. The presence of these small purple or red spots leaves a negative, lasting impression of the phlebotomy procedure with the patient. Any form of temporary or permanent disfigurement must be avoided, so be sure to remove the tourniquet in a timely manner and keep pressure on the site as long as necessary to stop the bleeding.

Question: What causes petechiae and what can stop it?

_____

_____

_____

Figure 4-7   Follow these steps for proper tourniquet application.

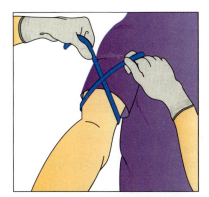

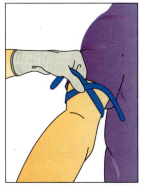

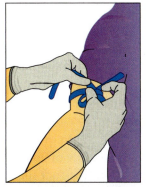

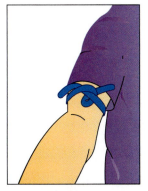

(a) Position the tourniquet under the arm while grasping the ends above the arm and venipuncture area. The tourniquet should be 3 to 4 inches above the site.

(b) Cross the left end over the right end and apply a small amount of tension to the tourniquet.

(c) Using the right middle finger or index finger, tuck the left end under the right end.

(d) A loose end of the tourniquet will be pointing toward the shoulder and the loop will be pointed toward the hand.

Figure 4-8 The antecubital area of the arm is the most common site to perform venipuncture.

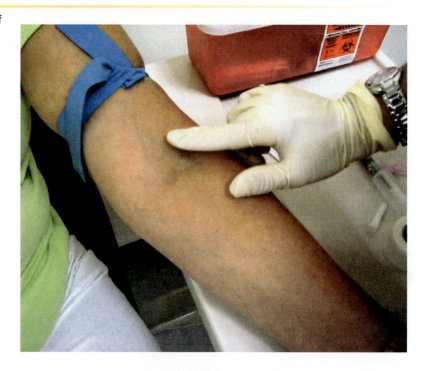

Selecting the Venipuncture Site

The most common area to perform a venipuncture is in the inside of the elbow, or antecubital area of the arm (see Figure 4-8). This is where the median cubital, cephalic, and basilic veins lie close to the surface of the arm (see Chapter 2, Figure 2-8, on page 41). Locate the median cubital vein, which is usually the largest and best-anchored vein, near the center of the antecubital area. Always examine this area first, because the easiest veins to collect from are located in the antecubital area of the arm. Patients generally have more prominent veins on their dominant arm. For example, if the patient is left-handed, look for a vein in the left arm first. You should check and palpate both arms before deciding on the site for the venipuncture.

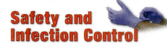

Safety and Infection Control

Prevent Choking

A patient should not be drinking, eating, or chewing gum during the phlebotomy procedure. Any foreign object in the mouth during phlebotomy could cause choking.

To help locate veins better, position the arm at a downward angle, using the force of gravity as an aid in making the veins more prominent. In addition, instruct the patient to make a fist, but not to attempt to pump the fist because this can cause hemoconcentration. The preferred way to increase the vein size, making the venipuncture easier, is to warm the site by using a warm, moist compress for 3 to 5 minutes, if time permits. Using plastic such as a plastic side of a blue pad or a plastic bag or gloves against the skin is

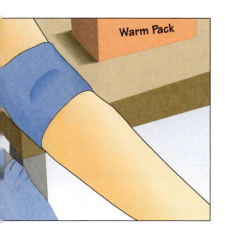

Warm Pack

Figure 4-9 The preferred way to increase bloodflow and make the venipuncture easier is to warm the site.

a good idea. This will dilate the veins and increase the bloodflow but keep the skin at the site from getting wet (see Figure 4-9).

While you are selecting the venipuncture site, explain to the patient the importance of holding the arm very still. Tell the patient that holding the arm still will reduce the discomfort of the venipuncture. If the patient moves during the venipuncture procedure, the needle will "tear" the vein and muscle, causing pain and damage to the venipuncture site. Additionally, if the patient moves during phlebotomy, the phlebotomist could miss the venipuncture site and fail to collect the blood specimen.

Palpating the antecubital area will help you determine the size, depth, and direction of the vein. Palpate the vein using the tip of the index finger. Select a vein that is large and does not roll from side to side or move easily. The larger the vein, the better for blood collection. It is common to feel for the bulge of the vein, but try feeling for the valley instead of the bulge. Try closing your eyes if you have trouble feeling a vein. Closing your eyes will enhance your sense of touch. An appropriate vein for venipuncture will bounce and have resilience to it. A vein that exhibits **sclerosis,** or feels hard and cordlike (i.e., lacks resilience), should be avoided. A vein that feels hard tends to roll easily and should not be used for a venipuncture.

Troubleshooting

Hematoma

A hematoma, or mass of blood caused by leakage of blood into the tissues, will occur if the tourniquet is left on the arm too long. A hematoma (a raised area forming near the site) will occur if the tourniquet is left on the arm after the needle is taken out. Blood will leak into the tissues from the venipuncture site. A hematoma will occur if the needle has gone through the vein or if the bevel of the needle is not inserted fully into the vein. If you notice the formation of a hematoma, release the tourniquet, pull the needle out, and apply firm pressure at the site. If the patient complains of discomfort, apply ice to the hematoma.

Question: After venipuncture you notice a raised, painful area on the venipuncture site. What should you do?

_____

_____

_____

Troubleshooting

Hemoconcentration

Hemoconcentration is a rapid increase in the ratio of blood components to plasma. Hemoconcentration can be caused if the patient vigorously pumps (rapidly opens and closes) the fist, the phlebotomist leaves the tourniquet on for longer than one minute, or the tourniquet is simply too tight. Hemoconcentration happens long before it is noticed by the patient, usually in three to five minutes. Pain, pressure, or a "falling asleep" sensation can occur during hemoconcentration. Hemoconcentration should be avoided

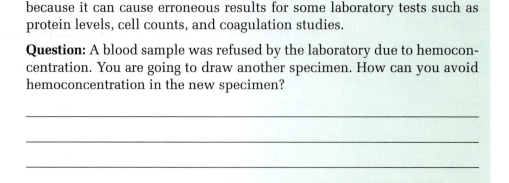

because it can cause erroneous results for some laboratory tests such as protein levels, cell counts, and coagulation studies.

Question: A blood sample was refused by the laboratory due to hemoconcentration. You are going to draw another specimen. How can you avoid hemoconcentration in the new specimen?

_____

_____

_____

Carefully select the vein to be used for venipuncture. Try to mentally visualize the location of this vein and note the position of the vein in reference to hair, skin creases, or a mole. Once a vein has been selected, release the tourniquet to lessen the chance of causing hemoconcentration in the venipuncture area during the cleansing procedure. Mental visualization of the vein will help you to locate the vein after releasing the tourniquet. You must clean the skin before venipuncture, and having a landmark will help you locate the selected site again. An experienced phlebotomist may choose to apply the tourniquet, clean the area, and perform the venipuncture all in one step. This should only be done if the venipuncture site is dry before the blood is collected and the tourniquet stays on the arm less than one minute. Meeting these two conditions is difficult, especially for the new phlebotomist.

As you recall from Chapter 2, arteries should never be selected for a routine venipuncture procedure. Arteries are usually located much deeper beneath the skin than veins, so you probably will not encounter them. The phlebotomist needs to be aware of the differences between an artery and a vein, however. You can feel the difference between an artery and a vein because arteries are more elastic and have thicker walls than veins. In addition, arteries will pulsate when palpated. Tendons can also be mistaken for veins. However, they do not have the elastic feel and are hard to the touch.

If no acceptable vein is available in the antecubital area of both arms, remove the tourniquet and check the wrist or hand for acceptable venipuncture sites (see Figure 2-9 in Chapter 2 on page 41). Veins in the back of the hand may be used only if necessary. A winged infusion set or butterfly with pediatric tubes may be used for this site. Hand veins are delicate and small; therefore the smaller vacuum tubes such as the pediatric ones may be best for this procedure. The air in the tubing of the butterfly set can decrease the amount of blood obtained. Thus a smaller needle and adapter are preferred over the butterfly set. Veins in the hand tend to move or "roll." To avoid this, ask the patient to help position the hand downward to hold the vein taut. This can be accomplished by placing the thumb of the non-sticking hand about one inch below the site of insertion. Apply pressure on the vein and push slightly downward. Foot and ankle veins should be used only as a last resort and can be used only if a written order from the licensed practitioner is obtained.

Special Considerations When Selecting a Venipuncture Site

The venipuncture site should be free of lesions, abrasions, and scar tissue. Never select an arm that is **edematous,** or full of swelling. Because of the fluid buildup in the tissue, the vein will not be prominent. If you apply a tourniquet, it will not be effective in showing the vein and it will leave an indentation on the arm. If the patient has an IV in place, perform the venipuncture procedure on the other arm. Venipuncture should never be performed above the IV site. If a specimen is collected above an IV, the fluid given through the IV will affect the laboratory results. However, if no other site is available, drawing a blood sample below an IV site is acceptable. The arm on the side of a mastectomy (breast removal) should also be avoided because of the potential harm to the patient due to lymphostasis. **Lymphostasis,** or lack of fluid drainage in the lymph system, commonly occurs in patients who have had lymph nodes removed, such as during a mastectomy.

Special Considerations for Children

It is good practice to ask a child to help with the phlebotomy procedure. A child can hold a tube adapter, a piece of gauze, or even a bandage. This will help take the child's mind off the procedure and make the phlebotomy process easier for you. If specimens from children are routinely collected, it is a good idea to have special bandages or stickers available as rewards for good helpers. Being honest and direct with the child is best; however, the child should be allowed to view the needle for as short a period as possible to help reduce anxiety.

Special Geriatric Considerations

The process of aging presents physical problems that can be challenging for the phlebotomist. Physical conditions such as arthritis and diseases that cause tremors will require the phlebotomist to take extra time with the patient. In addition, sensory impairment, such as loss of hearing or vision, requires further patient preparation. Hearing loss may require the phlebotomist to repeat the instructions, and loss of eyesight may require careful guiding of the patient to the phlebotomy chair.

The skin of an elderly person is thinner, therefore making the venipuncture more difficult. The phlebotomist must hold the skin down or taut so that the vein does not move or roll. Additionally, as we age the muscles become smaller, so the angle of venipuncture should be shallow during needle insertion.

Special Considerations for Patients with HIV or Hepatitis

It is understandable for the phlebotomist to worry about patients with infections such as HIV and hepatitis. Sometimes these patients are in denial or angry, therefore they may be hostile or combative when having their blood drawn. This can cause a great concern for the phlebotomist. It is essential for the phlebotomist to use all personal protective equipment when placed in this situation. If the phlebotomist feels an accident could occur due to the patient being irate and creating an unsafe work environment, the phlebotomist must report the patient to his or her supervisor before drawing blood. An occupational exposure should be avoided.

Special Considerations for Psychiatric Patients

The challenges presented by psychiatric (mentally ill) patients may test your technical skills as well as your interpersonal skills. Psychiatric patients may have a hard time remaining calm and still during the procedure. They can be combative, scared, or anxious due to fear of the unknown. Or they may simply not understand the procedure that is taking place due to their frame of mind or medication. Psychiatric patients can have a difficult time grasping an idea or concept, thus making your job as a phlebotomist more difficult. Evaluate the patient carefully for any signs that the process of blood collection could be difficult. If you have a concern, have another phlebotomist or staff member assist you when obtaining specimens from psychiatric patients.

Cleansing the Venipuncture Site

Cleaning or washing the venipuncture site with an antiseptic (alcohol pad) helps prevent microbial contamination of the specimen and the patient (see Figure 4-10). However, it will not sterilize the site. The recommended antiseptic is 70% isopropyl alcohol, the antiseptic used in alcohol pads. Cleanse the site by using **concentric circles.** Start the circular motion at the center of the selected site and move outward in an ever-widening circle. To remove surface dirt you must apply sufficient pressure. If the site is especially dirty, repeat the procedure (with a new alcohol pad) to ensure that the site is thoroughly cleaned. Allow the alcohol to dry completely. It is the drying action of the alcohol that dries out the cells of bacteria. Never blow on the site or fan it to hasten the drying process.

Patient Education & Communication

Pediatric Patients

Discretion and common sense must be used at all times, but especially when dealing with children. The phlebotomy procedure will usually be frightening to a child. Never lie to a patient (child or adult) by telling them, "This will not hurt." Even the most smoothly performed phlebotomy procedure will cause momentary discomfort to the patient. For children it is best to keep them talking to distract them and then quickly proceed with the procedure. Usually a parent is present and can assist with the phlebotomy procedure and reassure the child. For most purposes the consent of a parent is enough informed consent to proceed with the procedure.

Figure 4-10 When cleaning the venipuncture site **(a)** use an alcohol prep pad with firm pressure to clean the venipuncture site. **(b)** Move outward in concentric circles.

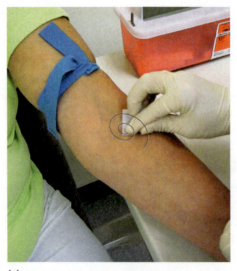

(a)

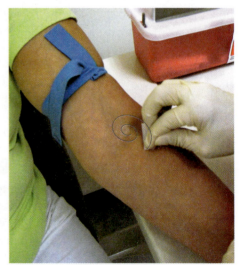

(b)

Troubleshooting Use of Alcohol

If the venipuncture is attempted before the alcohol is allowed to dry, it can result in a burning sensation for the patient when the needle enters the skin. If wet alcohol enters the needle and becomes mixed with the specimen, the specimen will be hemolyzed and the laboratory results will be affected. In addition, it is the drying action of the alcohol that dries out the bacteria on the skin.

Question: Why should the venipuncture site be allowed to air dry?

_____

_____

_____

Checkpoint Questions 4-2

1. What steps are involved in preparing for the venipuncture procedure?

_____

_____

_____

2. What types of patients or conditions may require special considerations during blood collection?

_____

_____

_____

 Answer the questions above and complete the *Preparing for Venipuncture* activity on the Student CD under Chapter 4 before you continue to the next section.

4-3 Performing the Venipuncture

Now that you have the patient prepared for the venipuncture procedure you are ready to perform the venipuncture. You will need to verify the site, insert the needle, collect the specimen, and remove the needle. You will also need to know what to do if the venipuncture attempt is unsuccessful.

Verifying the Venipuncture Site

After reapplying the tourniquet, have the patient make a fist again to help you visualize the vein. Using your dominant hand, pick up the venipuncture assembly with the thumb on the top of the tube adapter and the fingers underneath. Remove the needle cover and visually inspect the needle tip. Look for obstructions, imperfections, or barbs along the needle shaft and needle tip. If any abnormalities are noted, you must replace the needle with

Figure 4-11 Position the needle with the bevel up and inspect it carefully before insertion.

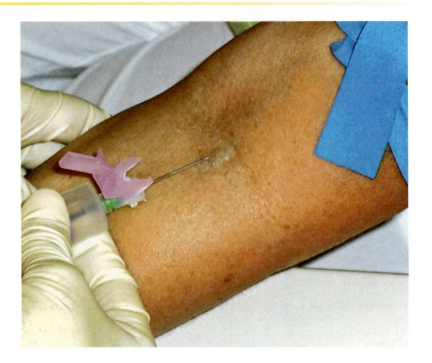

a new sterile needle. While inspecting the needle note the bevel area of the needle and position the bevel up. Positioning the needle bevel upward will make it easier to insert the needle into the skin and will cause less pain to the patient (see Figure 4-11).

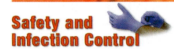

Safety and Infection Control

Keep the Needle Sterile

The needle must not touch anything. If you touch or lay the unsheathed needle down for any reason, it becomes contaminated and a new needle must be used in its place.

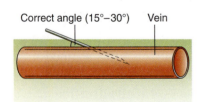

Correct angle (15°–30°)   Vein

Correct insertion technique
(Blood flows freely into needle)

Figure 4-12 Insert the needle at a 15- to 30-degree angle.

Inserting the Needle

Use the thumb of your nondominant hand (the one without the needle) to pull the skin taut one to two inches below the needle insertion site while gently grasping the patient's arm. Holding or grasping the patient's arm will help anchor the arm and the vein. Pulling the skin taut will also help anchor the vein, keeping it from rolling or moving during insertion of the needle. For a successful venipuncture, line the needle up with the vein. If the needle position is the same as the vein position, successful venipuncture is more likely. Make sure the bevel of the needle is facing you, or pointed up, and in the same direction as the vein. To avoid startling the patient, warn the patient when you are about to draw blood. You could say, "There is going to be a stick now." You might also want to remind the patient to remain very still during the procedure. Using one smooth motion, insert the needle into the skin at a 15- to 30-degree angle. You will feel a decrease in resistance or a slight "pop" when the needle enters the vein (see Figure 4-12). The first sign of a successful venipuncture is blood in the evacuated tube, after the tube is completely inserted.

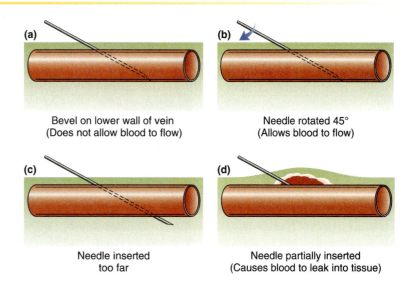

Figure 4-13 Various needle positions include **(a)** the bevel against a vein wall, **(b)** the needle rotated 45 degrees, **(c)** the needle inserted too far, and **(d)** the needle partially inserted, causing a hematoma.

(a) Bevel on lower wall of vein
(Does not allow blood to flow)

(b) Needle rotated 45°
(Allows blood to flow)

(c) Needle inserted too far

(d) Needle partially inserted
(Causes blood to leak into tissue)

If the Venipuncture Is Not Successful

Failure to obtain a blood specimen may be remedied by various techniques. Insufficient vacuum in the tube can cause blood collection failure. There is no way to check tube vacuum before a venipuncture. Always keep an extra tube close at hand. If the needle position appears correct, a loss of tube vacuum is the most likely reason for failure of blood to appear in the tube. Replace the defective tube with another tube. If you still cannot obtain a blood specimen, reposition the needle by pulling back slightly. The bevel may be against the wall of the vein, stopping the bloodflow. If no blood flows, advance the needle slightly further into the vein because the needle may not have penetrated the vein wall (see Figure 4-13). If the needle is over halfway into the patient's arm, pull the needle back slowly until it is positioned inside the vein and blood begins to enter the tube. The needle can penetrate too far into the vein and exit beyond the vein wall to the other side. Applying the tourniquet too tightly can also stop bloodflow, so try releasing the tourniquet slightly. Finally, probing the site with the needle is not recommended and is extremely painful to the patient. Probing is much different than repositioning the needle. During probing the needle position is changed. It is better to try another site rather than to probe. If available, you may want to use an instrument, such as a venoscope, to visualize the vein (see Figure 4-14). The battery operated venoscope uses LED (light emitting diodes) lights to illuminate the subcutaneous tissue and highlight the veins that absorb the light.

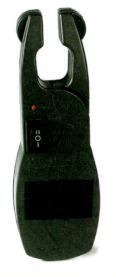

Figure 4-14 A venoscope is a special light that can be used to visualize the veins for venipuncture.

Collecting the Specimen

It is important to hold the venipuncture assembly steady during the entire tube-filling procedure (see Figure 4-15). Grasp the flange of the tube holder with your index and middle fingers. Use your thumb to push the tube to the end of the adapter. If the needle is properly positioned in the vein, blood will flow freely into the evacuated tube. During the filling process, care should be taken to keep the needle as stable and motionless as possible. Some phlebotomists release the tourniquet once collection has started; others wait until the entire draw is finished to ensure that there is no **venous reflux** (backflow). Either way is permissible. However, many practicing

Figure 4-15 Hold the assembly steady while collecting the blood. Do not leave the tourniquet on for more than one minute.

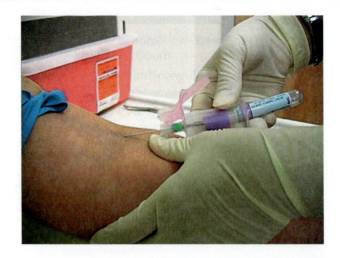

phlebotomists would suggest releasing the tourniquet when the last tube is about one-half full. A tourniquet should not be left on the patient during specimen collection for longer than one minute. If bloodflow stops once you release the tourniquet, it is permissible to reapply the tourniquet and leave it on for three or four tubes (approximately one minute). The reapplying of a tourniquet is difficult without help. If you are using an elastic strip you would need both hands to reapply it.

Collection tubes are filled according to the order of draw outlined in Chapter 3. Continue filling the evacuated tube until the bloodflow stops inside the tube. Bloodflow will stop once the vacuum is gone from inside the evacuated tube. The amount of vacuum inside each tube has been designed so that a consistent amount of blood is drawn into each evacuated tube. Overfilling an evacuated tube is not possible unless the stopper is removed and blood is added. This is sometimes done when drawing multiple samples with a large syringe. Underfilling an evacuated tube is possible if it is removed from the assembly before it is completely filled. When an evacuated tube is full, the proper dilution or mixture of additive to blood has been achieved.

To change tubes during collection, brace the thumb against the flange of the holder and use a pulling motion while removing the tube (see Figure 4-16). Next, place the new tube into the holder and gently push the tube

Figure 4-16 Hold the needle steady while removing and replacing tubes during the blood collection.

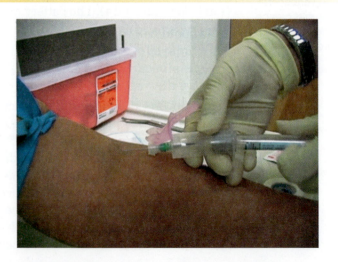

all the way into the needle. Care should be taken not to move or pull the needle out of the patient's arm during tube changes. Collect or fill all necessary tubes for tests requested. Mix them immediately the recommended number of times as determined by the additives inside each tube. Most tubes with additives need to be inverted gently 8 to 10 times (see Figure 4-17).

Troubleshooting

Handling Syncope

During phlebotomy, **syncope** (fainting) can occur. The symptoms to look for in the patient include heavy perspiring, pale skin, and shallow or fast breathing. Following this, the patient experiences drooping eyelids, rapid and weak pulse, and finally unconsciousness. If the patient does have a syncoptic episode, immediately remove the tourniquet and needle, then call for help. Apply pressure to the venipuncture site. Do not attempt to handle this situation alone, and don't leave the patient. Position yourself in front of the phlebotomy chair or next to the bedside to block the patient from falling or sliding out of the chair or bed. Lower the patient's head and arms by placing both the head and arms between the patient's knees. If a sink is near the patient, wipe the patient's forehead and back of the neck with a cold compress.

Question: Your patient looks pale and starts to slide down in the chair during blood collection. What should you do?

_____

_____

_____

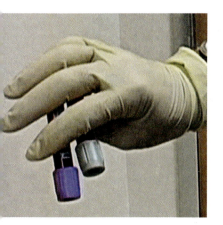

Figure 4-17 When necessary, mix the specimen by inversion.

HIPAA, Law & Ethics

Number of Attempts

Each health care facility has its own policy regarding the number of times a phlebotomist should attempt to get a blood specimen. Generally, two is the maximum number of times you should stick a patient. If you are unsuccessful after two tries, you need to ask for assistance. Repeated, unnecessary needlesticks can cause damage to the patient. You can be held liable if you fail to follow your institution's policies and patient injury occurs.

Removing the Needle

Remove the last tube from the holder and, with your other hand, fold the gauze into half or quarters, then gently place it directly over the area where the needle enters the skin. Do not apply pressure on the gauze or skin because this will cause pain to the patient before and during needle removal. Using one smooth motion, withdraw the needle from the patient's arm. Engage the safety mechanism right before or right after the needle

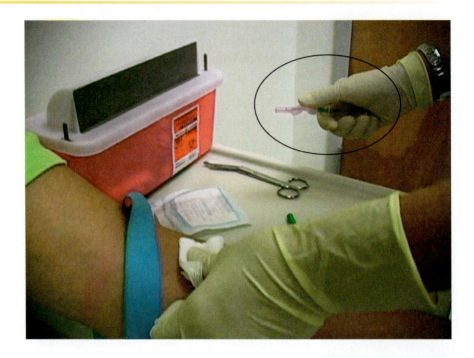

Figure 4-18 The safety mechanism should be engaged immediately.

is withdrawn, depending upon the type of needle used (see Figure 4-18). Immediately apply gentle pressure to the site for three to five minutes or until bleeding stops. The arm should remain straight or not bent at the elbow to prevent ecchymoses. **Ecchymosis** is bruising or discoloration caused by the seeping of blood underneath the skin.

The patient should be instructed not to disturb the platelet plug that is forming at the venipuncture site. It is common for a patient to want to bend the arm after needle removal, but tell the patient not to bend the arm upward. Bending the arm may cause bruising. The patient should not pick at, blot, or wipe the venipuncture site. You may ask the patient to apply pressure for you. Check later to see if the bleeding has stopped.

If pressure is not applied to the venipuncture site after removing the needle, a hematoma will form. If the tourniquet is left on and the needle is removed, blood will be forced out of the hole the needle left into the surrounding tissue and into the layer of skin, resulting in a hematoma. Some patients may be on blood thinners and will bleed for longer than other patients. Do not leave the patient if bleeding has not stopped.

Checkpoint Questions 4-3

1. What is the first sign that the venipuncture is successful?

_____

_____

_____

_____

2. Which is less likely and why: an underfilled evacuated tube or an overfilled evacuated tube?

_____

_____

_____

_____

Answer the questions above and complete the *Performing the Venipuncture* activity on the Student CD under Chapter 4 before you continue to the next section.

4-4 After the Venipuncture

Once all tubes are filled and the needle is safely removed, you will need to perform a few more steps to complete the phlebotomy procedure. Your first responsibility is to the patient. Make sure the patient is comfortable and holding pressure on the venipuncture site (see Figure 4-19). Then proceed to disposing of the needle and labeling the specimen (see Figure 4-20). You will also need to apply a bandage and transport the specimen before you are done.

Patient Education & Communication

Do Not Discuss the Tests

The patient may ask about the blood tests being drawn. Patients usually want to know how much blood will be drawn or the purpose of the tests the health care provider requested. It is best to state that the tests are routine tests the physician has ordered. If the patient needs more information regarding the tests, suggest that he or she speak with the physician. The phlebotomist should not discuss the tests with the patient. If the phlebotomist were to tell a pregnant woman that an RPR for syphilis (a sexually transmitted disease) was to be drawn, for example, and this was the first she heard of it, imagine the anxiety and panic this woman might feel, not to mention the doubt created toward her husband or significant other.

Disposing of the Needle

It is proper to dispose of the needle and adapter as one piece. It is not acceptable to unscrew the needle from the adapter to discard it. Drop both articles into the sharps container at one time. Do not place your hand inside the sharps container. Keep your opposite hand and arm back and away from the contaminated needle.

Sharps containers should be made of a puncture-proof material and display the biohazard symbol. Please pay close attention when disposing of sharp materials. Never overfill the sharps container. Once it is two-thirds full, place the lid on tight and place in a biohazard box for disposal or

Figure 4-19 Have the patient apply firm pressure to the venipuncture site.

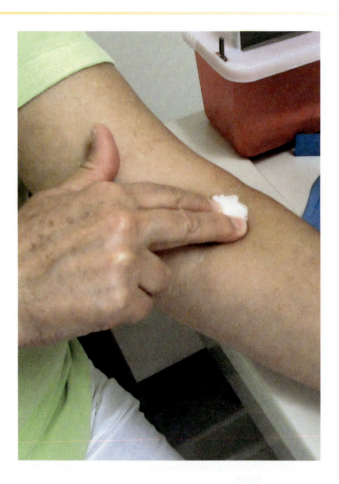

Figure 4-20 Carefully dispose of the needle and adapter in the sharps container.

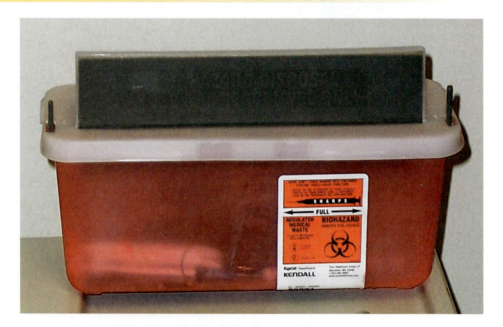

follow the specific policy at your facility. Remember to check the sharps container before the blood collection procedure so you are not left with a contaminated needle and no place to discard it. The sooner a contaminated needle enters the sharps container, the less chance of accidental needlestick.

Figure 4-21 Properly labeled collection tubes include the patient's full name, medical record number, date, time of collection, and your initials.

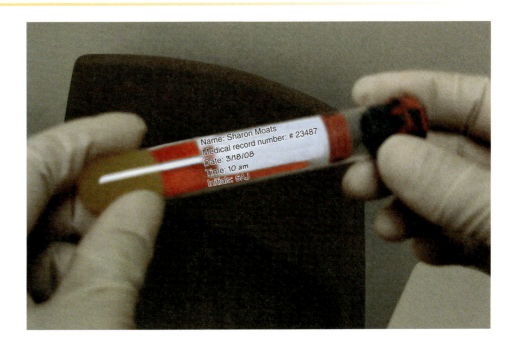

Name: Sharon Moats
Medical record number: # 23487
Date: 3/18/08
Time: 10 am
Initials: SAJ

Labeling the Specimen

Remember that all specimens must be labeled properly before leaving the patient's room or blood collection area. Label all specimens immediately using computer-generated labels or write with a permanent marker on the tubes (see Figure 4-21). Required information consists of the patient's full name, the patient's hospital number or identification number, the time of collection, the date, and your initials. Make sure you write the time of collection on the computer-generated labels and initial them. Your initials or code number must be present in case there is a question about the specimen, so the medical laboratory technician or technologist will know who to ask. The actual time of collection is critical in fasting specimens and in the monitoring of therapeutic drug levels. For therapeutic drug monitoring, peak or **trough levels** (collected when a serum drug level is at its lowest, usually immediately before the next scheduled dose) may need to be collected.

Always label the blood tubes after the blood is drawn. This is done for several reasons. A tube may have lost its vacuum, in which case the label is wasted because it is difficult to transfer most computer labels. You may not be able to obtain a sample and need another phlebotomist to attempt draw and it would have the wrong phlebotomist's name on the label. At an inpatient facility, sometimes blood tests are canceled or the patient has been discharged by the time you reach the floor.

Another reason to not pre-label is that you may be interrupted by a STAT request while away from the lab drawing blood. This request requires that you respond to immediately and postpone drawing another patient's blood until the STAT blood specimen is drawn. The only safe way to collect specimens is to label the specimen at the time of collection.

To prevent mislabeling, do not label before or after you leave the patient, only at the time the specimen is collected. Improperly labeled specimens can lead to serious patient complications. Imagine that a potassium level is drawn on a patient who has a very low level, yet the specimen bears the label of another patient. The patient whose blood was drawn may then receive unnecessary potassium supplements while the other patient may not get the needed potassium replacement therapy. Both patients' medical care would be greatly compromised, and the mix-up may even result in death. Proper labeling can be a matter of life or death.

Preventing Bleeding

A patient may say the bleeding has stopped, leave the phlebotomy area, and remove the arm gauze, then return a few moments later with blood dripping down the arm. What has happened is that the venipuncture wound appeared to be closed and the bleeding stopped, but movement of the arm caused it to open back up. This would not happen if proper procedures were followed. For this reason, a bandage is applied for most outpatient venipuncture. Advise the patient to apply pressure for several minutes before taking off the bandage or gauze. In addition, caution the patient not to use the venipuncture arm to push off with, open doors, or lift heavy objects such as a purse.

Applying the Bandage

Check the patient's arm to verify that bleeding has stopped. At a minimum, bleeding usually stops after three minutes. This is approximately the time it takes to properly label the specimen tubes and dispose of the used needle. To hold the folded gauze in place, apply an adhesive bandage or paper tape over the folded gauze. The patient can remove the bandage after 15 minutes. If the patient is allergic to bandages or tape, either have the patient apply pressure for a while longer, apply paper tape over the gauze, use a roller gauze completely around the arm, or apply a Coban® (elastic) dressing (see Figure 4-22). If the patient is elderly and the skin tends to tear when tape or bandages are applied, the phlebotomist should hold pressure a little longer to ensure that bleeding has stopped. To prevent injury, do not use tape on anyone with thin or fragile skin. Notify the patient's health care provider so he or she can recheck the venipuncture site. The patient should never remove the pressure until the bleeding has stopped, not just on the surface but at the vein level. Bleeding may no longer be present on the skin, but this does not mean a clot has completely formed in the vein. Once a clot has formed, no bandage is actually needed. Although a bandage is recommended in most cases, it is the patient's decision as to whether one is applied. Remember, small bandages are not recommended for small children who may choke on or swallow them.

Properly put away and dispose of all other supplies and equipment used in the venipuncture procedure. Place the unused evacuated tubes back in their proper places. Dispose of used alcohol pads, dirty gauze, trash from the needle assembly, and adhesive bandages in the trash receptacle. Remove and dispose of gloves in the biohazard trash receptacle and wash your hands. Thank the patient and leave the phlebotomy area as it was before the procedure.

If an inpatient specimen was collected, replace the bedrail in the same position as it was before the procedure. Move any other items back into place you may have moved for the venipuncture procedure. Dispose of nonsharp,

Figure 4-22 Apply a bandage to the site to avoid disturbing the platelet plug and causing further bleeding.

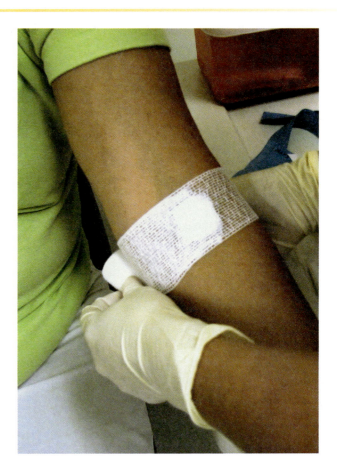

noncontaminated items in the patient's trash can, but any tubes or glass slides must be disposed of properly in the laboratory. Thank the patient and, if the door was closed when you entered, close the door when you exit.

Transporting the Specimen

Transport the specimens to the laboratory in a timely manner. In some laboratories the outpatient phlebotomy area is part of the whole laboratory, so transporting requires only going to the next room. However, sometimes the phlebotomy area is in a different part of the building, so transportation becomes more important. Some medical facilities use pneumatic tube systems or a dumbwaiter to expedite transporting specimens to the laboratory. Some laboratory tests, such as erythrocyte sedimentation rate in hematology, must be set up or performed within one hour of collection. Other laboratory tests must be centrifuged, or separated, within a specified amount of time. Ideally, the specimen should be taken to the lab in 45 minutes and centrifuged within one hour. Standards recommend a limit of two hours between collection and separating serum or plasma by centrifuge. If you are unsure of specimen requirements, look them up in the procedure manual. If the blood is not taken to the laboratory in the necessary length of time, the test results will be inaccurate.

Outpatient facilities present a different situation with regard to transportation of laboratory specimens. Usually a courier service transports the specimens from the collection facility to the reference laboratory. Specimens

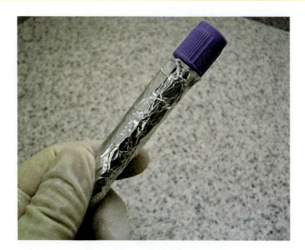

Figure 4-23 Special handling procedures may involve wrapping tubes in foil or placing the tube in a cup of ice-water mixture.

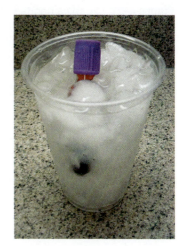

may need to be processed at the outpatient facility before transportation to the reference laboratory. Specimen processing is covered in detail in Chapter 5.

You may be required to follow special handling procedures for the specimens drawn. Special handling applies to specimens that are to be kept warm, protected from light (wrapped in aluminum foil), or put into an ice-water mixture immediately (see Figure 4-23). Table 4-1 presents a list of common laboratory tests that require special handling. These requirements apply from the time of collection to the specimen processing.

Checkpoint Questions 4-4

1. What should be done immediately before or right after removing the needle?

   _____

   _____

   _____

   _____

   _____

2. When should the blood tubes be labeled?

   _____

   _____

   _____

   _____

   _____

 Answer the questions above and complete the *After the Venipuncture* activity on the Student CD under Chapter 4 before you continue to the next section.

TABLE 4-1 Common Laboratory Tests That Require Special Handling

Laboratory Test	Special Handling
Acid phosphatase	Deliver to lab within hour Separate, freeze serum after clotting
Adrenocorticotropic hormone (ACTH)	Place in ice-water mixture**
Alcohol, blood	Use antiseptic other than alcohol prep pad
Ammonia	Place in ice-water mixture
B_6 (vitamin)	Protect from light
B_{12} (vitamin)	Protect from light
Beta-carotene	Protect from light
Bilirubin, total or direct	Protect from light
Catecholamines	Place in ice-water mixture
Clot retraction	Incubate in 37°C until clotted
Cold agglutinins	Warm tube, incubate in 37°C until clotted Separate immediately after clotting
Complement, C4	Separate, freeze serum after clotting
Complement, total (CH50)	Let clot in refrigerator Separate immediately, freeze serum
Complement, total (CH100)	Let clot in refrigerator Separate immediately, freeze serum
Gastrin	Place in ice-water mixture
Gentamicin	Label peak or trough
Glucose tolerance	Label tubes with time interval
Human leukocyte antigen (HLA-B27)	Do *not* refrigerate or freeze Record date and time collected
Lactic acid	Place in ice-water mixture
Parathyroid hormone (PTH)	Place in ice-water mixture
pH/blood gas	Place in ice-water mixture
Porphyrins	Protect from light
Prostate-specific antigen (PSA)	Deliver to lab within hour Separate, freeze serum after clotting
Prostatic acid phosphatase	Deliver to lab within hour Separate, freeze serum after clotting
Pyruvate	Place in ice-water mixture
Thioridazine (Mellaril®)	Protect from light
Tobramycin	Label peak or trough
Vancomycin	Label peak or trough
Vitamin A	Protect from light*

*Protect from light = protect by wrapping the tubes in aluminum foil.
**Place in ice-water mixture = place tube in a cup with a mixture of ice and water.

4-5 Using a Butterfly Needle Set

The butterfly needle set, or winged infusion set, has been reported to be less painful to patients. However, the use of the butterfly needle set results in more accidental needlesticks. Thus, the butterfly needle set should only be chosen when a standard venipuncture cannot be performed. Butterfly needle sizes range from 21- to 25-gauge in diameter and ½ to ¾ inches in length (see Figure 4-24). Infants, children, and some adults have small veins that may require using a butterfly needle set with a syringe. If a smaller amount (less than 10 mL) of specimen is needed, a safety needle attached directly to a syringe will suffice. When a butterfly is used with evacuated tubes, the small or delicate vein can collapse, stopping the specimen collection process (this is referred to as a **collapsed vein**). A syringe does not have a vacuum, so the phlebotomist can control the amount of pressure applied to small or delicate veins. A luer adapter attaches the butterfly needle set to the syringe.

Performing the Venipuncture with a Butterfly Set

When performing a venipuncture using a syringe attached to a needle or butterfly needle set, follow the steps for routine venipuncture. However, you should be aware of some differences. Equipment setup includes selecting evacuated tubes needed for specimen transfer from a syringe. Place the evacuated tubes in the correct order of transfer into the collection rack. Collection tubes are filled from the syringe, referring to the specimen transfer order as outlined in Chapter 3 on page 62. Put all other necessary venipuncture equipment within an arm's reach before starting the procedure.

Next, remove the syringe from the sterile packaging and push the plunger in and out to ensure free and smooth movement during the venipuncture procedure. Before beginning, make sure the plunger is pushed completely in. Aseptically attach the syringe to a safety needle or butterfly setup. Make sure the plunger is pushed all the way in and perform the venipuncture procedure as described earlier in this chapter. Hold the syringe in the same manner as you would hold the tube holder. The first sign of a successful venipuncture is blood in the hub, or clear area, of the needle. Care must be taken when pulling the plunger back so you do not accidentally withdraw the needle from the arm. The barrel of the syringe

Figure 4-24 A butterfly needle set includes **(a)** a safety needle with butterfly wings, **(b)** connecting tubing, **(c)** an evacuated tube holder, and **(d)** evacuated tubes.

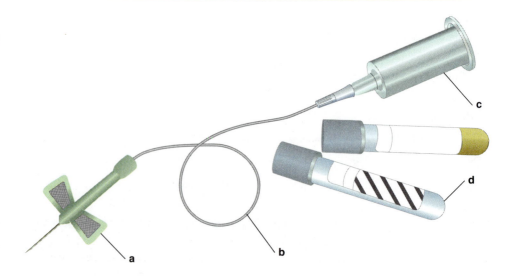

TABLE 4-2 Laboratory Tests Affected by Hemolysis

Severely Affected	Considerably Affected	Barely Affected
APTT—activated partial thromboplastin time	ALT—alanine aminotransferase	Acid phosphatase
AST—aspartate aminotransferase	ANA—antinuclear antibodies	Albumin
CBC—complete blood count	B_{12}, vitamin	Ca—calcium
K—potassium	Blood bank antibody screen	Mg—magnesium
LD—lactic dehydrogenase	Folate	P—phosphorus
PT—prothrombin time	Fe—iron	TP—total protein
	T4—thyroxine	

will fill with blood as you pull the plunger out. Complete the syringe collection in the same manner as routine venipuncture.

When using a syringe, care should be taken so that the specimen is not hemolyzed, which means the red blood cells are destroyed or broken apart. If the plunger is pulled back too hard or fast, the cells racing through the needle will be hemolyzed. These cells will rupture (break apart) and release their contents, resulting in a hemolyzed specimen that is unsuitable for most laboratory tests (see Table 4-2). Also, if the plunger is pulled back too hard, the vein may collapse. This is caused by the vacuum created by the syringe and the plunger.

Transferring the Specimen to Tubes

Immediately after removing the needle from the patient's arm, transfer the blood collected in the syringe to evacuated tubes using a blood transfer safety device (see Figure 4-25). Evacuated tubes are filled from the syringe in the

Figure 4-25 Using a syringe transfer device.

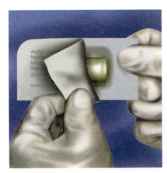

1. Peel off backing from transfer device.

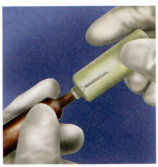

2. Insert syringe tip into hub and rotate syringe clockwise to secure.

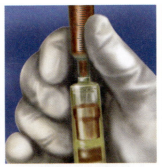

3. Hold the syringe facing down and push the evacuated tube into the holder. Do not depress the plunger of the syringe.

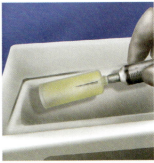

4. After removing the evacuated tube, discard the tube holder and syringe in an approved sharps container.

same order of the draw as outlined in Chapter 3. When using a blood transfer device you will need to first remove the needle from the syringe. Before removing the needle, make sure the safety mechanism is engaged so the needle is not exposed. Attach the device to the syringe and then insert the evacuated blood collection tube in the transfer device. Allow the blood to transfer using the vacuum in the tube. Do not depress the plunger as this may result in hemolysis. When the tubes are filled, dispose of the transfer device and syringe into the appropriate sharps container.

Using a Butterfly Needle Set with Evacuated Tubes

A butterfly needle set can be used with an evacuated tube adapter. Evacuated tube adapters come in two sizes, one for regular-size tubes and one for pediatric-size tubes. A butterfly needle set has tubing that attaches the needle to the evacuated tube adapter area. Tubes are pushed into the adapter in the same manner as in routine venipuncture. The whole butterfly set is disposed of in the same manner as a regular needle in the sharps container.

Disposing of a Syringe and Butterfly Needle Set

Extra care should be taken when disposing of a butterfly needle set. When the needle is removed from the arm, the needle tends to hang from the butterfly assembly tubing, exposing both the phlebotomist and the patient to a potential needlestick injury. Be certain to use the safety device. It should be employed immediately on withdrawal from the vein, and in some cases before the needle is withdrawn from the patient. Some safety devices have a hard plastic cover that snaps into place after withdrawing the needle. Other safety devices retract the needle into a special holder or safety device. A safety device should always be present and engaged as soon as possible after blood collection.

✔ **Checkpoint Questions 4-5**

1. When should a butterfly needle set be used and why?

   _____

   _____

   _____

   _____

2. What technique is used to move blood from a syringe to an evacuated tube?

   _____

   _____

   _____

   _____

Answer the questions above and complete the *Using a Butterfly Needle Set* activity on the Student CD under Chapter 4 before you continue to the next section.

4-6 Performing a Dermal Puncture

Dermal puncture is the blood collection technique of preference for infants and very small children. Because of a child's smaller size, it is difficult to locate a vein that is large enough to withstand the vacuum exhibited by evacuated collection tubes without collapsing. Children do not enjoy venipuncture and usually do not remain still for the length of time a venipuncture requires. Dermal puncture is employed if the test requested requires a small amount of blood. Venipuncture may be more difficult for infants and small children. In some cases, patients who are obese, elderly, or severely burned may have difficult veins to locate, making dermal puncture a possible alternative. Be certain to check the policy at your facility. Dermal punctures are not always acceptable for the laboratory test ordered. See Table 4-3 for a comparison of blood collection methods.

The blood specimen obtained during dermal puncture is a mixture of capillary blood, venous blood, arterial blood, and fluids from the spaces surrounding the tissues. Because of new and developing technology in laboratory instrumentation, most laboratory tests can now be performed on capillary blood. The most notable exceptions are blood cultures and erythrocyte sedimentation rate (ESR), because both of these tests require a relatively large

TABLE 4-3 Comparison of Collection Methods

Method	When to Use	Pros	Cons
Evacuated tube	Routine collection Whenever possible	Fast Relatively safe Best specimen quality Large collection amount possible	May not work with: small veins fragile veins difficult draws small children hand or foot
Butterfly assembly	Small veins Fragile veins Difficult draw Small children	Least likely to collapse vein Less painful for patient Least likely to pass through small veins	Syringe not as safe: tube transfer Specimen may be hemolyzed Not good for large amounts of blood Expense Increased risk of needlestick
Dermal puncture	Children Infants Elderly patients Oncology patients Severely burned patients Obese patients Inaccessible veins Extremely fragile veins Home testing by patient Procedure requiring capillary specimen only	Easy to perform Requires small amount of specimen	Not good for dehydrated patient Not good for patient with poor circulation Cannot collect for certain tests such as: blood cultures ESR

amount of blood. One drawback of a dermal puncture for the laboratory is the amount of blood collected. The small amount collected using dermal puncture usually leaves an insufficient amount of sample if the test requires a large amount of blood or needs to be repeated.

Preparing for Dermal Puncture

Many of the preparation steps for dermal puncture are the same as those for venipuncture. Before you begin the actual procedure you perform the following steps in the same manner as done with venipuncture.

- Acquire and examine the requisition slip.
- Greet and identify the patient.
- Explain the procedure.
- Verify any diet restrictions.
- Wash your hands.
- Put on gloves.

The main differences between venipuncture and dermal puncture are the site selection and equipment assembled (see Figure 4-26).

Selecting the Site for Dermal Puncture

The skin should be warm, pink, and free from scars, cuts, rashes, or bruises. The sites to consider for dermal puncture are the third and fourth fingers in

Figure 4-26 Equipment for dermal puncture.

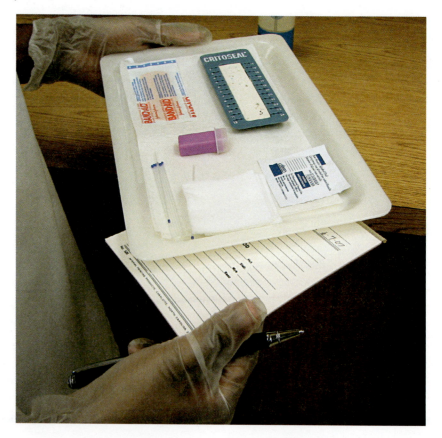

Figure 4-27 The dark areas indicate correct sites for finger and heel dermal puncture.

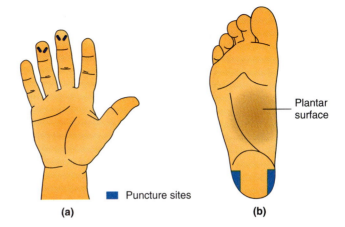

Puncture sites

Plantar surface

(a)   (b)

children and adults and the heel in infants (see Figure 4-27). For a finger puncture, do not use the thumb, pinkie, or pointer finger; they are poor choices, because the area is often too thick and callused. Always puncture across the grain of the fingerprint lines. Do not use the end or tip of the finger.

In infants of less than one year who are not walking, the heel is the recommended puncture site. Never perform a dermal puncture on a walking infant because of the potential for pain at the site. Examine the infant heel and choose the lateral surface for dermal puncture. Do not use the arch of the foot, the back of the heel, or the **plantar** area (bottom surface or sole) of the foot. If an infant has several old puncture sites, attempt to find an unused area. The site chosen for puncture should be well away from the area of the **calcaneus,** or heel bone. If the calcaneus is punctured, it could cause **osteomyelitis,** an infection of the bone. In premature infants, the calcaneus is less than 2.0 mm below the surface of the skin.

Troubleshooting **Crying Infant**

Excessive crying by an infant can cause an elevated leukocyte count. It takes 60 minutes for the leukocyte count to return to normal. Therefore, if an infant has just had a procedure (e.g., circumcision or vaccination) that resulted in excessive crying, you should wait 60 minutes before attempting blood collection.

Question: You are sent to the newborn nursery to collect blood from a newborn. When you arrive the infant is just being brought back from a circumcision. What should you do?

_____

_____

_____

For children and adults, the preferred site for dermal puncture is the **palmar** (palm side) surface of the finger. Usually the ring or middle finger of the nondominant hand is chosen. The dermal puncture site of choice is the sides of the fingertip. Slightly warming the finger with a warm cloth (or the heel with a heel warmer) will enhance bloodflow.

TABLE 4-4 Dermal Puncture Site Selection Summary

Recommended Areas	Areas *Not* Recommended
Heel; medial and lateral plantar surfaces	Back of heel, bottom of foot, arch of foot
Central fleshy area of third and fourth fingers	Callused finger (usually index finger), thumb, or pinkie
Across fingerprint lines	Along fingerprint lines
	Areas with visible damage or edema
	Sites previously used for dermal puncture

The finger to be punctured or cut for a dermal puncture should not be edematous. Edema is caused by a buildup of fluids, with the result that the specimen will contain an abnormal amount of **interstitial fluid** (fluid between cells and tissues), which will cause abnormal laboratory results. Look at the other hand to see if it is also edematous. If both hands are edematous, a venipuncture should be attempted.

Table 4-4 summarizes the recommended sites (and those to avoid) for dermal puncture.

Equipment for Dermal Puncture

The equipment needed for dermal puncture is the same with the exception of the puncture device and the collection containers. You will need a requisition slip, alcohol prep pad, gauze, gloves, adhesive bandage or tape, sharps container, computer label, permanent marker, or pen. As discussed in Chapter 3, you will need a safety dermal puncture device or lancet and microspecimen containers.

Microspecimen containers vary in size and shape. Some collection devices have a straw-like apparatus attached to the end. Capillary action—the force that causes fluids to rise into tubes with small diameters—helps these devices to fill with a pulling action. Some microcollection devices appear to fill by themselves once the end is brought near the drop of blood.

Safety dermal puncture devices have a blade or puncture point that retracts after the device is used. These safety devices operate differently depending upon the manufacturer and the location of puncture. Special devices have been developed for newborns and premature newborns and other devices are used mostly on children or adults. Devices are chosen based upon the age and size of the patient. Devices are frequently spring-loaded to control the depth and ensure the blade retracts to prevent accidental needlesticks.

Performing a Dermal Puncture

When a dermal puncture is performed, a cut is made into the layers of the dermal (skin) surface. The finger should be held in such a way that the skin is stretched tightly. For a finger dermal puncture, cut across the fingerprint line when you puncture the finger. Cutting across the fingerprint delivers the best possible flow and droplet formation for a dermal puncture (see Figure 4-28). If the cut is made between the fingerprint lines, the flow is less, and the blood tends to flow down the fingerprint, not forming drops.

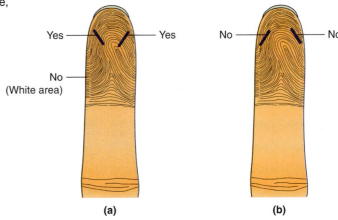

Figure 4-28 For a correct dermal puncture, **(a)** cut across the fingerprint; **(b)** do not cut in the same direction as the fingerprint.

Yes — Yes

No — No

No
(White area)

(a)   (b)

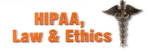

**HIPAA,
Law & Ethics**

Dermal Puncture Depth

Incorrectly collecting a dermal specimen can cause bone infection. This is especially true in infants. It could be considered malpractice if the calcaneus is punctured by mistake, creating a site for bacterial infection. This infection can lead to further infection of the surrounding bone, cartilage, and bone marrow. Puncture depth should never be greater than 2 mm.

Clean the finger with an alcohol pad and allow the finger to dry thoroughly. It is very important to allow the site to dry prior to collecting the dermal puncture specimen to prevent hemolysis of the blood due to contact with the alcohol. Apply slight pressure, then puncture the site with the properly selected safety device (see Figure 4-29).

Do not use spring-loaded devices designed for glucose monitoring when performing routine dermal puncture. These lancets produce a small puncture and only two or three drops of blood. Most microcollection containers need more than two or three drops to fill. After you have punctured the site, periodically gently squeeze and release, allowing for capillary refill. You should avoid milking the finger (a motion as if you were milking a cow) because it will not enhance bloodflow. In fact, milking may contaminate the specimen with interstitial fluid and it may cause hemolysis of the cells. Scraping the blood off the finger instead of allowing the blood to flow freely into the collection device also causes hemolysis. With scraping, the blood clots before it can be mixed with the anticoagulant in the microcollection device. The resulting clotted specimen is unsuitable for testing.

Use the device correctly. Check the directions. No matter which device or site (finger or heel) you use, dermal puncture will cause pain. It is better to make the first puncture deep enough, using the proper technique, than to have to puncture a second time to obtain sufficient blood.

Collecting the Capillary Specimen

Before collecting the blood into the microcollection device, wipe away the first drop of blood. This drop contains interstitial fluid and damaged tissue cells, which will contaminate the blood specimen. After the dermal

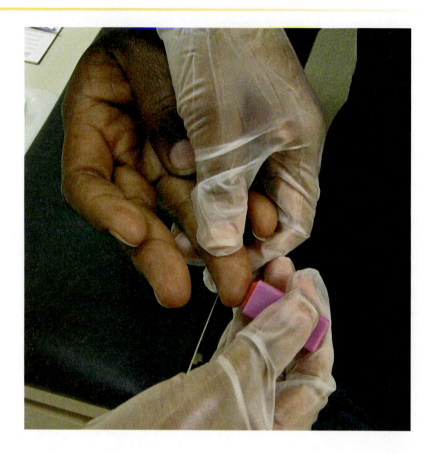

puncture, the capillary blood flows downward with the aid of gravity into the microcollection device. More than 0.5 mL of capillary blood can be collected by dermal puncture if the puncture is performed properly. At the puncture site, a drop of capillary blood forms. After the drop is formed, touch the open end (collection tube or scoop) of the microcollection device to it. The microcollection device will fill by gravity or capillary action, depending on the size of the collection area. Continue with an alternating pressure and release action until an adequate amount of blood is obtained. Keep the site down below the level of the heart to increase bloodflow. Correct dermal puncture collection involves allowing free-flowing drops to enter the collection device. The blood flows onto the tip and then down the walls of the microcollection device. As discussed in Chapter 3, these microcollection devices have an anticoagulant additive. If blood lodges or stops in the tip area, tap the device on a hard surface to mix the blood with the anticoagulant. This should cause the blood to flow down the side or wall. Most microcollection devices have a fill line. It is critical to collect to the fill line if an anticoagulant is inside the device.

Once an adequate amount of blood is collected, apply pressure to the puncture site with sterile gauze. Cap and label the microcollection device the same way as for routine venipuncture.

After the Dermal Puncture

Mix the specimens if necessary. Dispose of the contaminated safety lancet in the sharps container. Label the microcontainers and observe any special specimen handling instructions. Check the site of puncture and apply a bandage, when appropriate. Small children should not have bandages applied to their fingers because they have a tendency to put their fingers in their mouth and run the risk of swallowing or choking on the bandage. Collect and dispose of your supplies appropriately. Clean the area. Thank and dismiss the patient if appropriate. Remove your gloves and transport the specimen to the laboratory.

✓ Checkpoint Questions 4-6

1. Which patient would most likely have dermal puncture and why: a 10-month-old infant, a newborn, or an elderly patient?

_____

_____

_____

_____

_____

2. What are the two main differences between the dermal puncture and the venipuncture?

_____

_____

_____

_____

_____

Answer the questions above and complete the *Performing Dermal Puncture* activity on the Student CD under Chapter 4 before you continue to the next section.

Chapter Summary

- Patients must be properly identified for the blood collection procedure, including their name and another form identifier such as their birth date or medical record number. If one letter or number is different in either identifier, the blood should not be drawn unless proper identification is obtained.

- Prepare patients for blood collection by explaining the procedure, letting them know they can expect to experience pain from the needlestick. Position them in a supported seated or lying position.

- Tourniquets slow the blood to the site but if left on more than one minute can cause pain to the patient and hemoconcentration of the blood specimen.

- The venipuncture and dermal puncture sites are selected based upon their location and appearance. Venipuncture is typically performed in the antecubital area of the arm and dermal puncture is typically performed on the heel of an infant or third or fourth finger of an adult.

- Cleaning the site for dermal puncture most often requires the use of an alcohol prep pad, wiping in a circular motion from the center out. The site must dry thoroughly before the collection of blood.
- The specimen label includes the patient's full name, the patient record/identification number or birth date, date and time of the collection, and the phlebotomist's initials.
- The maximum number of times a phlebotomist should attempt blood collection is two.
- When you are unable to obtain blood during venipuncture, first change tubes in case the vacuum is lost from the first tube, then reposition the needle by pulling back slightly. Lastly you may want to loosen the tourniquet.
- A butterfly needle set should be the last resort when attempting blood collection; however it may become necessary in certain circumstances.
- Dermal puncture and venipuncture are similar procedures with the exception of the site of puncture and type of equipment used.

Chapter Review

Multiple Choice

Circle the correct answer.

1. You notice that a patient has just finished his breakfast when you arrive to collect his fasting blood glucose specimen. Which of the following should you do?
   a. Collect the specimen anyway since he has finished eating.
   b. Collect the specimen and indicate "nonfasting" on the requisition slip.
   c. Refuse to collect the specimen and fill out an incident report.
   d. Inform the patient's nurse; if the specimen should still be collected, write "nonfasting" on the label and requisition slip.

2. When is a phlebotomist allowed to perform a venipuncture on an ankle vein?
   a. Never
   b. When the patient has IVs in both arms
   c. During an emergency
   d. When all options are exhausted and the physician has given approval

3. The most important step in performing a venipuncture is:
   a. Removing the tourniquet before taking the needle out
   b. Drawing the correct amount of blood
   c. Inserting the needle in the vein properly
   d. Identifying the patient

4. No armband is present on an inpatient. What should the phlebotomist do?
   a. Leave and do not collect the specimen.
   b. Draw the blood specimen anyway.
   c. Ask the patient's nurse to put an armband on the patient.
   d. Go to the nurse's station and make an armband, then place it on the patient yourself.

5. The vein most frequently used for venipuncture is the:
   a. Brachial artery
   b. Cephalic
   c. Median cubital
   d. Saphenous

6. To produce a rounded drop of blood, finger punctures should be made:
   a. Before the alcohol is dry
   b. Across the fingerprint
   c. Along or on the fingerprint
   d. On the index finger

7. All of the following are situations in which an arm vein should *not* be used except:
   a. Both arms are edematous
   b. An IV is running in the patient's only arm
   c. Both arms are badly burned
   d. Both arms are strapped

8. When a patient develops syncope during a venipuncture, the phlebotomist should first:
   a. Lower the patient's head
   b. Immediately remove the needle and call for help
   c. Complete the venipuncture as quickly as possible
   d. None of the above

9. When cleaning the site for venipuncture you should perform all of the following except:
   a. Use 100% isopropanol
   b. Use 70% isopropanol
   c. Allow alcohol to air dry
   d. Rub the alcohol pad in concentric circles from inside out

10. In general, what is the maximum number of times you should stick a patient?
    a. One time
    b. Two times
    c. Three times
    d. Unlimited

11. What is the effect of warming the site prior to dermal puncture?
    a. It may cause hemolysis in the specimen.
    b. It increases bloodflow to the area.
    c. It makes the puncture less painful.
    d. It causes hemoconcentration.

12. The angle at which you enter the vein should be:
    a. Bevel up at a 15° angle
    b. Bevel up at a 45° angle
    c. Bevel down at a 15° angle
    d. Bevel down at a 45° angle

13. During a fingerstick collection, excessive milking can cause:
    a. Irritation at the site
    b. Excessive bleeding
    c. Contamination of the specimen with tissue fluid
    d. Contamination of the specimen with milk

14. During a venipuncture, if the area surrounding the vein begins to swell, you should first:
    a. Take the needle out of the arm
    b. Probe to get back into the vein
    c. Remove the tourniquet
    d. Finish collecting the specimens needed, then apply ice

15. Advancing the stopper of a collection tube past the mark or ridge on the adapter during equipment setup will:
    a. Cause hemolysis in the specimen collected
    b. Help ensure that the evacuated tube is working properly
    c. Make the venipuncture less painful for the patient
    d. Cause a loss of the vacuum in the tube

16. According to guidelines, the depth of a heel stick lancet should be no more than:
    a. 1 mm
    b. 1.5 mm
    c. 2 mm
    d. 2.4 mm

17. Why should the first drop of blood be wiped during a dermal puncture?
    a. To remove any interstitial fluid contamination
    b. To limit the amount of blood released
    c. To increase the amount of blood released
    d. To decrease the possibility of bloodborne pathogen transmission

18. What is the most serious error a phlebotomist can make?
    a. Inappropriate attire
    b. Inappropriate attitude
    c. Failure to identify a patient correctly
    d. Failure to inform the patient of what to expect

19. What will happen if a tourniquet is left on too long?
    a. Hemoconcentration
    b. Excess bleeding
    c. Site infection
    d. Specimen contamination

Ordering

20. Based on what you have learned in this chapter, put the following steps in order for performing a routine venipuncture by numbering them from 1 to 12 in the spaces provided.

    _____ a. Release tourniquet
    _____ b. Apply tourniquet
    _____ c. Explain procedure to patient
    _____ d. Wash hands and put on gloves
    _____ e. Label tubes
    _____ f. Anchor vein
    _____ g. Identify patient
    _____ h. Select and cleanse venipuncture site
    _____ i. Apply pressure to puncture site
    _____ j. Remove tube and mix
    _____ k. Introduce yourself
    _____ l. Insert needle into patient's arm
    _____ m. Remove the needle apparatus

Matching

Match each definition with the correct term. Place the appropriate letter on the line to the left of each definition.

21. _____ ecchymosis

22. _____ calcaneus

23. __a__ collapsed vein

24. _____ basal state

25. _____ peak level

26. _____ petechiae

27. __c__ plantar

28. _____ postprandial

29. __j__ hemoconcentration

30. __i__ fasting

a. Bruise caused by blood under skin

b. Metabolic condition after 12 hours of fasting and lack of exercise

c. The heel bone in the foot

d. An abnormal retraction of the vessel walls stopping bloodflow

e. After eating a meal

f. Pertaining to the sole of the foot

g. Specimen collected when the serum drug level is at its highest level, usually 15 to 30 minutes after administration

h. Minor hemorrhaging in underlying tissue

i. No food or liquids for 12- to 16-hour period

j. Increase in ratio of blood components to plasma

True or False

Write T or F in the blank to indicate whether you think the statement is true or false. Correct any false statements to make them true.

31. _____ Patient identification is a crucial step in obtaining a blood specimen.

32. __F__ STAT tests are usually obtained after your routine specimens.

33. _____ Vacutainer® tubes must be filled at least 75% to ensure accurate testing.

34. _____ When disposing of a used needle during a venipuncture procedure it is okay to unscrew the needle from the adapter and dispose of each separately.

35. _____ A venoscope is used to visualize the veins during phlebotomy.

What Should You Do?

In the space provided, describe what you would do in the following situations. Use critical thinking and troubleshooting. Be sure to include the reasons for your decisions.

36. Your patient, Mr. Tykodi, is not in his hospital room and you happen to see him in the family waiting area with his grandson. In the waiting area are several other patients with their families, several with young children. You approach Mr. Tykodi and tell him you are on the floor to draw his fasting blood glucose. He says, "Why not do it here in the sunshine?" What are your concerns about this situation? What would you do?

_____

_____

37. You are on the pediatric floor and Jennifer Burnham, a five-year-old girl, needs to have her blood drawn for a blood test. You enter her room and notice she is alone. You inform Jennifer you are here to take a blood test. She starts to cry and says, "Please, no more needles!" What would you do?

_____

_____

38. You are on your morning rounds on the fifth floor of the hospital. John Stallings in room 250 is scheduled to have blood work drawn. When you enter the patient's room, the patient identifies himself as James Stallings, but the armband says John Stallings. What is your next step?

_____

_____

_____

_____

39. You are going back to the lab to drop off your first set of specimens. As you begin to log the samples into the computer system, you find that you are missing a label on one of the specimens. What do you do?

_____

_____

_____

_____

40. You encounter a patient with very small veins. The patient has asked you to take your time and be patient with her. She has had several bad experiences in your office when it comes to blood collection procedures. The patient tells you that it is very difficult to obtain blood from her veins. You make one attempt and miss; you make another attempt and miss. What should be your next step after the second failed attempt to obtain a specimen?

_____

_____

_____

_____

Get Connected *Internet Activity*

Visit the McGraw-Hill Higher Education Online Learning Center *Phlebotomy for Health Care Personnel* Website at **www.mhhe.com/healthcareskills** to complete the following activity.

1. You are getting ready to start a position as a phlebotomist and will be doing lots of phlebotomy. Since you are going to be working by yourself most of the time, you would like to learn more about complications that can occur during this procedure and how to prevent or treat them. Search the Internet for more information about complications of venipuncture and make yourself a chart of various complications and what you should do.

Using the Student CD

Now that you have completed the material in the chapter text, return to the Student CD and complete any chapter activities you have not yet done. Practice your terminology with the "Key Term Concentration" game. Review the chapter material with the "Spin the Wheel" game. Take the final chapter test and complete the troubleshooting question. E-mail or print your results to document your proficiency for this chapter.

Specimen Handling and Processing

5

Learning Outcomes

Upon completion of this chapter, you should be able to:

- List requirements for special specimen handling procedures.
- Describe the technique required for collecting blood cultures.
- List the steps for Unopette® collection.
- Describe the procedure for performing a microhematocrit.
- Explain the collection process and procedure for making a peripheral blood smear.
- Discuss common point-of-care and CLIA waived tests.
- Explain the procedure for urine specimen collection and reagent testing.
- Identify safety requirements for operating a centrifuge.

Key Terms

aerobic	false negative
aliquoting	false positive
anaerobic	hematocrit
autoantibody	microhematocrit tube
bacteremia	normal flora
capillary tube	packed cell volume
chain of custody	pre-analytical error
cold agglutinin	septicemia
culture media	waived tests
differential	

5-1 Introduction

The process of venipuncture and dermal puncture involves more than just the collection of a sample of blood. Equally important is how the sample is obtained and how the sample is handled after the collection. Some samples require special handling and/or processing before and after the collection. In some cases other types of specimens may need to be collected. In addition, certain tests are done immediately at the point of care right after the collection of the specimen.

**Checkpoint
Question
5-1**

1. Other than collecting a blood specimen, what are some other duties relative to practicing phlebotomy?

_____

_____

_____

_____

_____

5-2 Special Specimen Handling Procedures

From the moment a blood test is ordered until it is tested various things can affect the test result and possibly cause an error. These things can occur before, during, or after the collection of the blood. Any error made before the actual analysis of the specimen is known as a **pre-analytical error.** Some errors can occur from the effects of light, heat, and contamination of certain blood tests. The way a specimen is collected and how it is handled are essential to an acceptable specimen and accurate results. For example, the collection process for blood cultures must be done in a manner that prevents contamination of pathogens from other sources than the blood. Forensic or legal specimens require accurate identification. Other tests may require heat, cold, or protection from light.

Blood Cultures

Blood culture samples are frequently requested for patients who have a high fever. The purpose of a blood culture test is to isolate microorganisms from the patient's blood sample. These microorganisms could be causing this fever. Strict aseptic technique is required for the collection of blood cultures. This requirement makes blood culture collection one of the most complicated phlebotomy procedures to perform correctly. Blood cultures must be obtained in special tubes or bottles that contain **culture media.** The culture media in these bottles enhance the growth of microorganisms. These tubes or bottles are usually larger and more cumbersome to handle than normal venipuncture tubes.

Some blood culture containers include an antibiotic removal device. In these devices a resin absorbs any antibiotic found in the specimen. These are typically used for patients who are on antibiotics at the time of culture and assist the physician in making a more accurate diagnosis (see Figure 5-1).

Figure 5-1 Aerobic and anaerobic blood culture bottles.

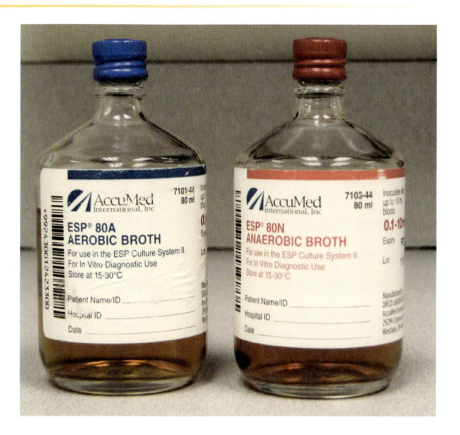

Safety and Infection Control

Accurate Blood Cultures

A pathogenic (disease-producing) organism in the blood is a serious condition that must be treated. However, sometimes the blood culture result indicates a pathogen is in the blood that actually occurred due to contamination during the collection procedure. When a blood specimen is contaminated with organisms that did not originate in the blood, this is a **false positive.** These organisms can get into the blood culture specimen due to:

- Inadequate cleaning of the puncture site
- Not allowing the cleaning agent to dry thoroughly
- Contaminated equipment or specimen containers
- Touching the puncture site after it has been cleaned

It is the responsibility of the phlebotomist drawing blood cultures to ensure that they are not contaminated during the procedure by strictly adhering to the blood culture procedure.

Blood is normally sterile, so the presence of microorganisms in the blood (**bacteremia**) can be very serious and result in death. **Septicemia** (the presence of pathogenic microorganisms in the blood with symptoms) will usually cause a person to have a fever. The largest number of organisms will be present in the blood right before a patient spikes a fever (has a sudden increase in temperature). The number of microorganisms causing the fever is still very small, so it is difficult to isolate them with only one sample. Therefore, a licensed practitioner will order the blood cultures to be drawn in sets of two or three. One sample, which includes two bottles or tubes, will be incubated (allowed time to develop or grow the existing microorganisms) as an **anaerobic** (living without oxygen or air) specimen, and the other sample will be incubated as an **aerobic** (living with oxygen or air) specimen. Each subsequent set should be obtained from different sites and/or at different time intervals. Blood cultures are usually requested STAT when a patient is spiking a fever, especially because antibiotics need to be administered to the patient and cannot be given until the samples are collected.

Blood cultures seek to identify the causative agent(s) responsible for the patient's illness, and this information assists the physician with prescribing medications, especially antimicrobial agents, and other treatments. Micro-organisms capable of producing diseases are called pathogens. The most common classifications of pathogens are as follows:

- Bacteria
- Viruses
- Fungi
- Protozoa

Many groups of microorganisms exist under each of the above classifications. If the causative agent isolated is identified as a bacteria, it can be from one of several groups of bacteria that exist. The blood culture helps identify the specific microorganism that causes the infection. For example, a culture would help differentiate between the bacteria *Streptococcus pyogenes,* which causes strep throat, and the bacteria *Streptococcus pneumoniae,* which is one agent responsible for pneumonia. Isolating the exact causative agent (microorganism) from the blood culture assists the physician in prescribing the antimicrobial that will work best to destroy the identified microorganisms.

Blood Culture Volumes and Collection

The volume of blood collected for a blood culture is critical. Each manufacturer of blood culture bottles or tubes has determined the optimum amount of blood sample needed to increase the chance of growing the microorganisms in the laboratory. Usually 8 to 10 milliliters (mL) per bottle or tube for an adult is sufficient. Lesser amounts are drawn on infants and children. See Table 5-1.

The amount of blood can have an impact on the test. For example, some bacteria such as *Escherichia coli* can exist in the blood in very low amounts, thus requiring a larger volume of blood to be drawn. If the volume is too low the bacteria are not seen in the culture, thus producing what is known as a **false negative** result.

TABLE 5-1 Recommended Blood Culture Volumes

Type of Patient	Aerobic Bottle Amount	Anaerobic Bottle Amount
Adult	8 to 10 mL	8 to 10 mL
Adult—low volume*	All obtained	None
Pediatric (based on weight)	2.5 to 10 mL	2.5 to 10 mL
Infant	0.5 to 1 mL	0.5 to 1 mL

If 10 mL or less is obtained from an adult, place all of the blood in the aerobic bottle.

In addition to getting the correct amount in each blood culture container, you must be certain to draw from the appropriate site and in the proper sequence. As mentioned earlier, a typical blood culture order requires two bottles (one aerobic and one anaerobic). These two bottles can be drawn from the same site. With some patients, however, the physician may order "blood cultures × 2." This would require that four containers be filled. The blood can be collected at the same time but must be collected from two different sites. If two sites cannot be used then the phlebotomist must wait a period of time, between 15 and 45 minutes depending on the order, before collecting the second set of blood culture containers at the same site. Collecting "blood cultures × 2 two different sites" or even "blood cultures × 2 fifteen minutes apart" is frequently done to prevent a false negative result.

Blood Culture Site Cleaning Procedure

The actual collection of the blood sample for blood cultures is similar to routine venipuncture, with added steps to ensure that the skin is as clean as possible. Cleaning the venipuncture site is the most important part of the blood culture collection procedure. Once the venipuncture site is selected, release the tourniquet. Cleanse the site using aseptic technique and the appropriate antiseptic. The normal cleansing process involves swabbing the area with 70% to 95% alcohol prep or other cleansing agents such as 0.5% chlorhexidine gluconate, or benzalkonium chloride (Zephiran chloride). (See Figure 5-2.) Start in the center at the site of puncture and continue outward in concentric circles using firm pressure. The phlebotomist must not allow the strokes to go back toward the center area. Stroking back to the central area would bring contaminants toward the selected puncture site. If aseptic or sterile technique were not followed, normal skin surface microorganisms (bacteria), known as **normal flora,** would be introduced into

Figure 5-2 The blood culture site must be cleaned thoroughly using an approved cleanser such as 0.5% chlorhexidine gluconate to prevent a false positive test result.

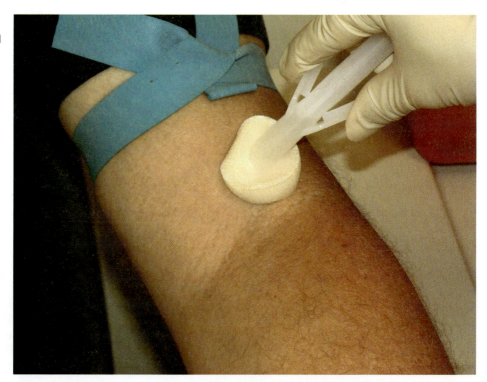

the blood culture sample and would interfere with the patient's results. The site cleaning process must be done with friction for at least 60 seconds to ensure the normal flora and contaminants are removed from the area. Once the site is cleaned, allow the cleansed area to air dry. The drying time gives the antiseptic time to kill the germs.

The primary purpose for cleaning the site is to reduce the number of normal flora at the selected puncture site. When using alcohol, once the initial cleansing area has air dried, you may be required to perform the same circular cleansing pattern, this time using a 2% iodine swab or applicator. If the patient is allergic to iodine, another cleanser is used. Check the policy at your facility and the current product directions to ensure the site is cleaned properly. Once the area is cleaned, it must not be retouched, even with a glove. If touched, the selected site would be considered contaminated and that would require repeating the entire cleaning procedure.

Patient Education & Communication

Cleaning the Blood Culture Site

As you are preparing a patient for blood culture collection, inform the patient about the procedure. Explain the importance of a sterile puncture and why you are cleaning the puncture area. Sometimes patients have a tendency to touch a venipuncture site, and this must be avoided during blood culture collections. If you were collecting a blood culture and the patient touched the site, you would have to clean the area again.

It is essential that the cleansing procedure is performed with great care. Patients requiring blood cultures are typically very sick. Since it takes 24 to 48 hours to get a preliminary result, if the procedure is not done correctly, the patient can lose critical treatment time waiting for the procedure to be repeated.

In many facilities, the tops of the blood culture bottles are also cleaned with iodine then wiped with alcohol. Some bottles from the manufacturer will have protective covers that will not require cleaning because they are sterile when opened. Check what is appropriate for the blood culture system your facility is using and follow the manufacturer's recommendations. Reapply the tourniquet, using extra care not to contaminate the cleansed venipuncture site.

Collecting Blood Culture Specimens

You can perform the venipuncture procedure with an evacuated system, syringe and transfer device, or a butterfly (winged) collection set. Once the tourniquet is reapplied, take extra care not to touch the clean site. If necessary, only touch at least an inch above and below the site. Do not touch the site even with a clean glove or the site cleaning will need to be repeated.

When a syringe is used you will need to make sure to obtain a syringe that will hold an adequate volume for both tubes. This is usually at least a 20 mL syringe for adults. Once you have obtained enough blood, remove the needle from the patient and engage the safety mechanism. Remove the covered needle and attach the syringe to a transfer device. Always fill the anaerobic bottle first in order to prevent air from entering this specimen. Next, fill the aerobic bottle and any other tubes required.

When using a butterfly setup the aerobic sample is drawn first in order to clear the air from the butterfly tubing before the anaerobic culture sample is drawn. If using a vacuum set you must be certain to have the correct type of tube holder so as to not allow culture media to accidentally enter the patient's blood. Review the manufacturer's directions.

After the blood is in the culture containers, label each with the date, time, and your initials. When doing more than one set of cultures, each set must also be labeled with the location of the draw, and the order of draw. For example, #1 L hand, and #2 R arm. If iodine was used, remove it from the patient's arm using a new alcohol prep pad to prevent absorption into the patient's skin. Remember, do not use iodine on a patient who has a possible allergy. Choose another approved cleanser.

Legal Specimens

Specimens of a legal matter require special handling. Blood and other specimens must be collected from a victim, suspect, or other person, dead or alive, involved in a legal matter. These specimens must be correctly identified and under the uninterrupted control of authorized personnel to ensure their validity. Accurately identifying a specimen and making sure it has not been altered or replaced is called establishing a **chain of custody.** This procedure is required for medicolegal issues such as evidence of rape as well as for drug tests for illicit drug use. If the chain between the victim and/or suspect and the specimen cannot be proved to have remained unbroken, the specimen must be considered invalid.

The first link in the chain of custody is collecting the specimen. If you are responsible for collecting the specimen, you must be sure the specimen is collected from the correct patient and that no one tampers with it. The chain-of-custody form (see Figure 5-3) must be completed correctly, and the patient may be required to sign or initial the form as well. Multiple copies of the form are used as a safeguard system. One copy, usually the original, accompanies the specimen in a sealed envelope. Another copy is attached to the outside of the envelope so that each person who handles the specimen can initial the form. A third copy is usually retained in the patient's file. These general procedures help maintain an intact chain of custody. Always refer to the procedure at your facility to make sure you are meeting all relevant requirements. More information about legal specimen collection is discussed in Chapter 6, "Special Phlebotomy Procedures."

Cold Agglutinins

Testing for **cold agglutinins,** or antibodies, is done for patients suspected of having conditions such as atypical pneumonia. Persons with atypical pneumonia are infected with *Mycoplasma pneumoniae*. People infected with Mycoplasma pneumoniae can produce **autoantibodies** (antibodies to yourself). These antibodies (immunoglobulins) attack something within your own body as if it were foreign.

Cold agglutinins react with red blood cells at temperatures lower than body temperature, which has a normal range of 97.6°F to 99.6°F (36.5°C to 37.6°C). The cold temperature reaction is the principle of the laboratory test for atypical pneumonia. After a blood sample is drawn, it begins to cool, or drop below body temperature. At temperatures lower than body

Figure 5-3 Each person handling a legal specimen must complete and sign the chain-of-custody form.

LABORATORY CHAIN-OF-CUSTODY FORM (SAMPLE)

Submitter:

(Complete Sections 1 and 2 before collection and document transfer of samples/evidence in Section 3.)

Section 1

Investigator name:		Date submitted:
Agency:		Agency case no.:

Address:			
City/County:		State:	ZIP code:
Phone no.:	Fax no.:	E-mail:	
Emergency contact:		Phone no.:	

Submitter: (Print name):	Agency: Telephone: ( ) -	Date:

Section 2

Sampling site:		Site address:
Collected by:	Date collected:	Agency:

Submitter description: Include the number of containers, identification number(s), and a physical description of each sample submitted for testing. {Relinquish sample(s) on page 2.}

Submitter comments:

Lockbox evidence seal number:

Section 3

Chain of custody: Persons relinquishing and receiving evidence: Provide signature, organization, and date/time to document evidence transfers. (Start with Box Number 1 below.)

Relinquished by (submitter)	Organization	Date/time	Received by	Organization	Date/time
1.			2.		

Relinquished by	Organization	Date/time	Received by	Organization	Date/time
3.			4.		

Relinquished by	Organization	Date/time	Received by	Organization	Date/time
5.			6.		

temperature, cold agglutinins in the serum attach to red blood cells, causing clumping. Collection tubes for cold agglutinins are red-topped tubes that contain no additives. Tubes must be prewarmed by placing them in a container of hot water or other warming device before collection and kept warm throughout the process. Tubes are usually placed in an incubator in the laboratory, set at 37°C (98.6°F) for 30 minutes. Care should be taken to keep the sample at 37°C (98.6°F). Failure to keep the sample warm will result in erroneous laboratory results. Cold agglutinin test samples must be kept at body temperature until the serum can be separated from the cells, which must be done within one hour. Routine venipuncture procedures are followed, with the noted addition of the warmed collection tube.

Chilled and Light-Sensitive Specimens

As mentioned in Chapter 4, some specimens must be chilled or covered immediately after collecting. Tests such as arterial blood gases, ammonia, and lactic acid require chilling. Blood collected for these tests will be placed in a container of ice and water. Specimens may even need to be collected in a chilled evacuated tube. Other tests are sensitive to light and will need to be covered in foil or placed in a special container to protect them from light. Blood tests such as a test for bilirubin require protection from light. This test is commonly performed on newborn infants. Refer to the policy at your place of employment to determine what special handling must be done for each blood test you will be collecting.

Checkpoint Questions 5-2

1. List three critical steps to perform during a blood culture.

_____

_____

_____

_____

_____

2. What one test requires a heated tube? An ice-water mixture? Darkness or protection from light?

_____

_____

_____

_____

_____

Answer the questions above and complete the *Special Specimen Handling Procedures* activity on the Student CD under Chapter 5 before you continue to the next section.

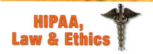

HIPAA, Law & Ethics

Follow Facility Protocol

It is the responsibility of a phlebotomist to make sure that the appropriate tube is used for each ordered specimen. Carelessness can cause inaccurate results that will adversely affect patient outcomes and definitely compromise patient care. The phlebotomist must follow the established protocol required for special collection procedures, including equipment and handling. If you are unfamiliar with a specific test, refer to the procedure manual available in the laboratory or ask for assistance. If you have any doubt about the test or procedure, you are ethically responsible for acquiring all needed explanations about a procedure prior to performing it. Patients have a right to quality health care performed by competent health care workers.

5-3 Unopette® Procedure

A Unopette®, manufactured by Becton Dickinson, is a popular type of microcollection device. The disposable device consists of a plastic reservoir and a pipette. The reservoir contains a premeasured volume of reagent for laboratory hematology tests such as a CBC. The most common tests using a Unopette® collection device include white blood cell count, red blood cell count, platelet count, hemoglobin, and RBC fragility. The pipette is a thin-walled, glass capillary tube that is attached to a plastic holder. The reservoir contains a specific reagent and the pipette is a specific size based upon the test being performed. The pipette is designed to collect the proper amount of whole blood for the reagent in the reservoir. So you must use the correct pipette with the correct reservoir or the test result will be incorrect. See Figure 5-4.

To open the Unopette®, place the reservoir on a flat surface. Puncture the diaphragm in the neck of the Unopette® reservoir with the capillary pipette shield. With a twisting motion, remove the pipette shield from around the pipette.

Figure 5-4 Parts of a Unopette®. The Unopette® system consists of a micropipette, a reservoir, and a pipette shield.

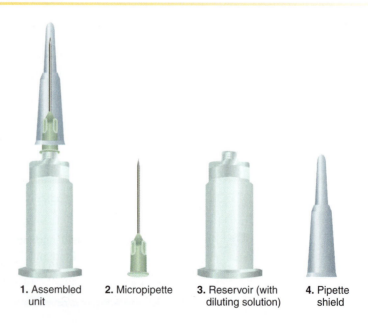

1. Assembled unit
2. Micropipette
3. Reservoir (with diluting solution)
4. Pipette shield

Figure 5-5 These steps illustrate the Unopette® procedure.

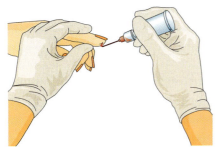

(a) Collect the specimen with the Unopette® pipette.

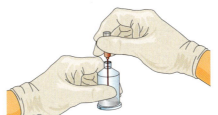

(b) Carefully squeeze the reservoir to mix the specimen.

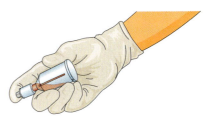

(c) Place a finger over the reservoir and mix by inversion.

Using a dermal puncture blood specimen, fill the capillary pipette with the blood sample. The pipette will stop filling automatically when the blood reaches the neck of the pipette. Carefully wipe the outside of the pipette with gauze and take extra care not to touch the end of the pipette. Gauze touching the end of the pipette will have a spongelike effect, causing loss of some of the blood sample from inside the pipette and thus resulting in erroneous laboratory results. Squeeze the reservoir slightly to remove the air, but do not expel any fluid. Maintain slight pressure on the reservoir and transfer the sample to the reservoir by inserting the filled pipette into the reservoir opening. Place your index finger over the opening of the overflow chamber. Maintain pressure until the pipette is securely in the reservoir neck. Release the reservoir pressure, then release the finger placed over the pipette. Negative pressure will draw the blood sample into the diluent in the reservoir.

To rinse the inside of the capillary pipette, carefully squeeze the reservoir several times. Do not squeeze the sample or diluent out of the top of the pipette. Place your gloved index finger over the opening and gently invert several times to mix the sample with the liquid inside the reservoir. Figure 5-5 illustrates the Unopette® system and procedure.

Troubleshooting **Unopettes®**

If part of the sample comes out of the top of the reservoir while mixing a Unopette®, some of the patient specimen can be lost. Insufficient quantity of specimen would result in erroneous patient results. You should recollect the sample from the patient.

Question: Why do you think losing part of the sample will cause inaccurate results?

_____

_____

_____

After collecting the Unopette® specimen, label it in the same way as you would label an evacuated tube. Transport the Unopette® to the appropriate laboratory section immediately.

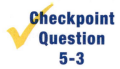
1. What is the Unopette® and what are its two parts?

_____

_____

_____

_____

 Answer the question above and complete the *Unopette® Procedure* activity on the Student CD under Chapter 5 before you continue to the next section.

5-4 Measuring Microhematocrit

Microhematocrit tubes are used for measuring a **hematocrit** (Hct or Crit), or **packed cell volume** (PCV). This disposable, narrow-diameter pipette has a colored red band around one end that indicates it is a sodium heparin–coated tube. See Figure 5-6. Microhematocrit tubes, or **capillary tubes,** are very slender, making them prone to breakage. A broken sharp edge can cause a break in the phlebotomist's glove and skin and consequently exposure to blood. To provide for safety, one type is a capillary tube made of plastic and another type is glass wrapped in plastic. As you will recall from Chapter 3, capillary tubes are filled by capillary action, which occurs when blood flows freely into the tube without suction.

To begin the hematocrit procedure, perform a dermal (capillary) puncture. Wipe away the first drop of blood with gauze. Using red-tipped capillary tubes, touch the tube to the edge of the drop of blood without touching the skin. In some cases, the capillary tube is filled from a tube of venous blood or a syringe. When filling the microhematocrit tube, air bubbles must

Figure 5-6 Capillary tubes may be colored at one end and are made of glass with plastic covering or plastic.

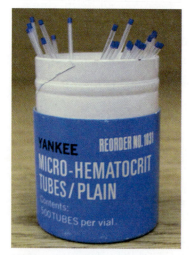

(a) Plain glass tubes

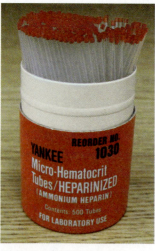

(b) Heparinized glass tubes

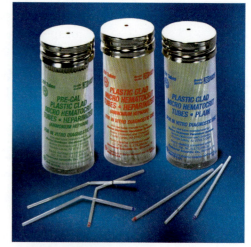

(c) Plastic tubes

not be allowed to enter the tube. Air bubbles in the microhematocrit tube can cause erroneous results. Fill two capillary tubes three-quarters full. The rate of filling can be increased or decreased by tilting the tube. However, do not remove the tip of the tube from the blood source with the tube lower than the blood. This will allow air to enter. Keep the tube horizontal or tilted upward during the filling process. Wipe excess blood off the outside of the capillary tubes with gauze. Hold the tube horizontally to prevent blood from leaking out of the tube.

Once a microhematocrit sample has been obtained, the capillary tube is usually sealed. The manufacturer's directions must be followed carefully to avoid tube breakage. Seal the end of the capillary tube that was not used to collect the specimen by embedding the clean end in a clay sealant designated for this use. Be careful not to lose any blood from the tube (see Figure 5-7). Improper sealing of the capillary tube will cause a decreased hematocrit reading. This decrease is a result of blood loss during centrifugation. Some microhematocrit tubes are self-sealing and do not require this puttylike sealant.

Because microhematocrit capillary tubes are fragile and too small to attach patient labels, place them in a separate tube for labeling and transporting the blood sample back to the laboratory. Attempts to label these small capillary tubes can result in breakage of the tubes, loss of the sample, and potential injury to the phlebotomist. Balance the microhematocrit tubes in the microhematocrit centrifuge with the clay ends facing outward

Figure 5-7 One end of the capillary tube may need to be sealed to prevent blood from leaking out of the tube.

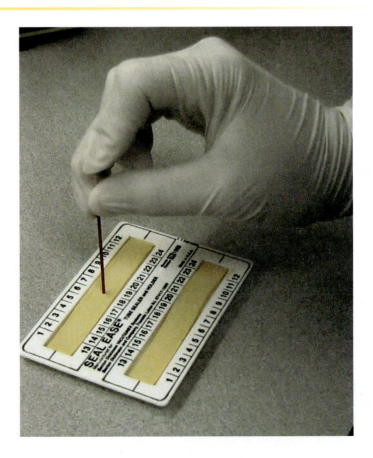

Figure 5-8 **(a)** Microhematocrit centrifuge. **(b)** When loading a microhematocrit centrifuge make sure that tubes are directly across from each other with the sealed end pointing to the outside.

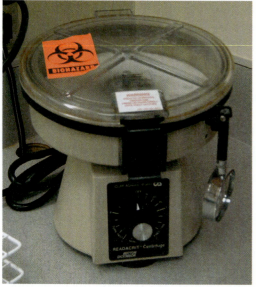

(a)

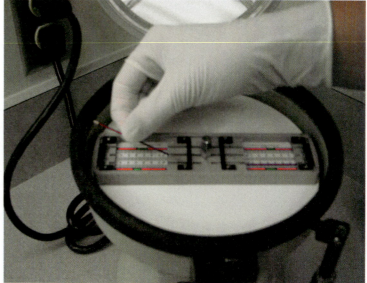

(b)

(see Figure 5-8). Tighten the head cover on the centrifuge and close the lid. Turn the microhematocrit centrifuge on for the appropriate time according to manufacturer instructions. The hematocrit is determined by using a microhematocrit-reading device. The two values of the microhematocrits (one from each tube) should match within two percent.

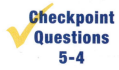

Checkpoint Questions 5-4

1. What is done to prevent air from getting into a capillary tube?

_____

_____

_____

_____

2. What is done to prevent leakage of blood from a capillary tube?

_____

_____

_____

_____

 Answer the questions above and complete the *Measuring Microhematocrit* activity on the Student CD under Chapter 5 before you continue to the next section.

5-5 Peripheral Blood Smears

A blood smear is for the microscopic examination of blood. Venous blood (blood from a vein collected in a tube) or capillary blood (blood collected by dermal puncture) may be used to prepare a blood smear. A blood smear can also be prepared by applying blood directly from the finger to the slide. The CBC (complete blood count) differential test utilizes a blood smear. Some of the most valuable information about a patient's health can be obtained through a well-made peripheral blood smear. A **differential** is a hematology test performed by a technician using a stained monolayer blood smear. The technician (using a microscope) examines and counts the different types of white blood cells as described in Chapter 2. In addition, the technician estimates the number of both platelets and white blood cells, determines red blood cell size and shape, and looks for any other blood abnormalities. Blood smears are also used to diagnose malaria and hematological disorders such as anemia and leukemia.

The Blood Smear Procedure

The "wedge" method is the most common technique for making blood smears. The blood smear should be made from fresh, uncoagulated drops of blood. Assemble the equipment needed for a dermal puncture or obtain a tube of uncoagulated blood. At least two clean glass microscope slides are needed to perform a blood smear. If performing a dermal puncture, wipe away the first drop of blood using a piece of gauze. Squeeze the punctured area to create a free-flowing drop of blood.

If you will be using a venous sample, check the specimen for proper labeling, carefully uncap the specimen tube, and use wooden applicator sticks to remove any coagulated blood from the inside rim of the tube or use a safety transfer device. Touch the tip of a capillary tube to the blood specimen either from the patient's finger or the specimen tube. The tube will take up the correct amount through capillary action. Pull the capillary tube away from the sample, holding it carefully to prevent spillage. Wipe the outside of the capillary tube with a sterile gauze square.

With the slide on the work surface, hold the capillary tube in one hand and the frosted end of the slide against the work surface with the other. Apply a drop of blood to the slide, about ½ inch from the frosted end. Place the capillary tube in the sharps container. Pick up the spreader slide with your dominant hand. Hold the slide at approximately a 30- to 35-degree angle. Place the edge of the spreader slide on the smear slide close to the unfrosted end. Pull or back up the spreader slide toward the frosted end until the spreader slide touches the blood drop. Capillary action will spread the droplet along the edge of the spreader slide.

Allow the blood drop to spread almost to the edges of the spreader slide. With one light, smooth, fluid motion, push the spreader slide toward the other, clear end of the slide until you come off the end, maintaining the 30- to 35-degree angle. On the bottom flat slide will be a thin film of blood in the general shape of a bullet or tongue. Allow the smear to air dry before staining. Figure 5-9 shows the steps in the wedge blood smear procedure.

It is important that most of the drop is spread out onto the glass slide. The smear will be thick at the drop end and thin at the opposite end. A good

Figure 5-9 Steps in the wedge blood smear procedure.

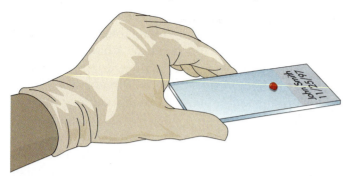

(a) Apply a drop of blood to the slide about ½ inch from the frosted end.

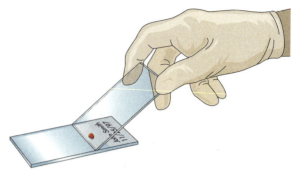

(b) Hold the spreader slide at a 30° to 35° angle. Pull the spreader slide toward the frosted end until it touches the drop of blood.

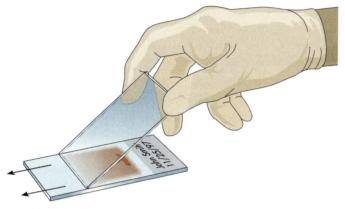

(c) When the drop covers most of the spreader slide edge, push the spreader slide back toward the unfrosted end of the smear slide.

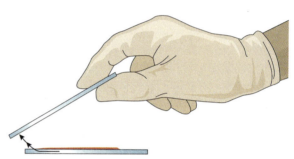

(d) Lift the spreader slide away from the smear slide, maintaining a 30° to 35° angle. The smear should be thicker on the frosted end of the slide.

Figure 5-10 A correctly prepared blood smear should be smooth in appearance without irregularities and should have feathered edges.

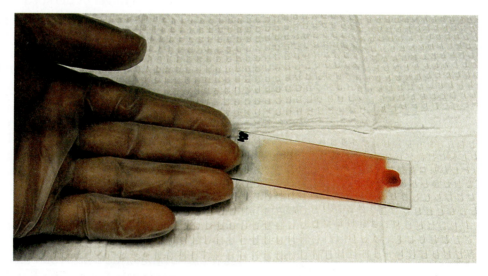

quality smear will be slightly rounded (see Figure 5-10). The blood smear should not touch the edges of the glass slide and should be smooth in appearance, with no irregularities, streaks, or holes. When the smear is held up to light, it will display a rainbow in the thin, "feathered" edge. Table 5-2 enumerates the criteria to ensure quality blood smears.

TABLE 5-2 Criteria to Ensure Quality Blood Smears

- Glass slides must be clean and free of chipped edges.
- The drop of blood should be about 2 mm in diameter.
- The smear should be made immediately after placing the blood on the slide.
- The spreader slide should be at a 30° to 35° angle.
- The pushing motion should be smooth and fluid.
- The smear should be allowed to air dry.
- The smear should cover two-thirds to three-fourths of the length of the slide (approximately 1½ inches).
- The smear should have a "rainbow," feathered edge.
- The smear should not touch any edge of the slide.

Checkpoint Question 5-5

1. Name at least three qualities of a good blood smear slide.

_____

_____

_____

_____

 Answer the question above and complete the *Peripheral Blood Smears* activity on the Student CD under Chapter 5 before you continue to the next section.

5-6 Point-of-Care Testing (POCT)

Point-of-care testing (POCT), or near-patient testing, is designed to reduce health care costs while enhancing patient care. These tests involve the collection of a sample followed by its immediate testing on an instrument at the patient's side. The purpose of POCT is to reduce the turnaround time for test results. POCT instruments are typically portable, internally calibrated, easy-to-use, self-contained devices that are operated with minimal training. The instruments are designed to make the performance of the test less dependent on the technical skill of the operator. Depending upon the health care environment, these tests are usually performed by a phlebotomist, nurse, patient care technician, or medical assistant.

Some of the POCT blood tests include glucose, hemoglobin, sodium, potassium, chloride, bicarbonate, ionized calcium, cholesterol, blood ketones, blood gases, hemoglobin A1C, and coagulation studies such as prothrombin time (PT), activated partial thromboplastin time (APTT), and activated clotting time. Other tests include urine dipstick, urine pregnancy tests, HIV salivary assay, guaiac (stool test for blood), and Strep A (throat culture screening).

POCT tests typically require a small amount of blood from a dermal puncture. However, each instrument is specific for the type of test, thus the type and collection requirements of the specimen are dependent upon the manufacturer's recommendations. All POCT instruments should be calibrated on a regular basis. The method of calibration is as individual as the test performed. Calibration and testing procedures are found in the manufacturer's directions. Regular calibration and instrument checking must be documented in a log book at the facility where you are employed.

POCT testing is done at various types of health care facilities. At in-patient facilities the clinical laboratory professionals provide oversight for quality of testing, regulatory compliance, method validation, accuracy checks, testing procedures, staff training, and technical support to areas or units performing testing.

For POCT to be at a location without a clinical lab, the only type of tests done are **waived tests.** CLIA regulations define waived tests as simple laboratory examinations and procedures that are cleared by the federal government for home use; that employ methodologies that are so simple and accurate that erroneous results would be negligible; or that pose no reasonable risk of harm to the patient if the test is performed incorrectly. A Certificate of Waiver must be obtained at these facilities.

Laboratories that function under a Certificate of Waiver must submit to random inspections and investigation, if indicated. Though waived tests are simple to perform and interpret, they may have serious consequences if done incorrectly. Patient care decisions are often made based on the outcome of waived tests.

In order to help ensure quality testing procedures and reduce patient error, the Clinical Laboratory Improvement Advisory Committee (CLIAC) has made several recommendations for good practice in a Certificate of Waiver laboratory. These recommendations include laboratory management considerations and testing procedures before, during, and after the test.

Laboratory Management and Personnel

- Designate the person who will be responsible for laboratory supervision. This person is usually a physician or someone with enough laboratory experience to make decisions about testing.
- Follow all applicable federal, state, and local regulations.
- Perform waived tests only.
- Follow manufacturer's instructions in the package insert.
- Do not make modifications to the instructions.
- Allow random inspections by authorized agencies such as the Centers for Medicare and Medicaid Services (CMS).
- Establish a laboratory safety plan that follows OSHA guidelines.
- Have a designated area that has adequate space and conditions.
- Have enough personnel in the lab and train them appropriately.
- Have written documentation of each test performed.

Before the Test

- Confirm written test orders.
- Establish a procedure for patient identification.
- Give patients pre-test instructions and determine whether they have followed these instructions.
- Collect specimens according to package insert instructions.

- Label specimens appropriately.
- Never use expired reagents or test kits.

During the Test

- Perform quality control testing as indicated in the package insert.
- Correct any problem discovered during quality control testing before testing patient samples.
- Establish a policy for frequency of control testing.
- Carefully follow all test-timing recommendations.
- Interpret test results using product inserts as a guide.
- Record test results according to your office policy.

After the Test

- Report test results to the physician in a timely manner.
- Follow package insert recommendations for follow-up or confirmatory testing.
- Follow OSHA regulations for disposing of biohazardous waste.
- Participate in quality assurance assessment programs:
  - Internal assessment—Perform routine, in-house testing to ensure the accuracy of a test.
  - External assessment—Voluntary inspection of your facility by an outside agency.

There are various POCT instruments (see Figure 5-11). One common point-of-care test is the blood glucose monitor. Instruments are available from different manufacturers. A POCT glucose determination allows the health care provider almost continuous monitoring of a patient's blood glucose inside and out of the health care facility. Changes in blood sugar can be handled immediately. Patients tend to be more compliant when they obtain immediate results. Testing provides the opportunity for better regulation of the patient's medication and condition.

Figure 5-11 **(a)** Glucometer; **(b)** hemoglobinometer; and **(c)** infectious mononucleosis, Strep A, and hCG urine pregnancy tests are common waived tests.

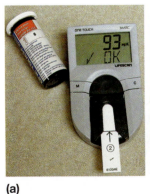
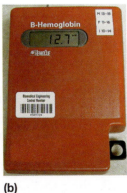
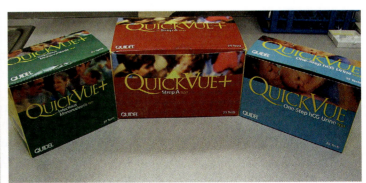

(a)   **(b)**   **(c)**

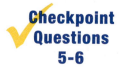
1. Name at least three point-of-care blood tests.

   _____

   _____

   _____

   _____

   _____

2. What is the advantage of POCT?

   _____

   _____

   _____

   _____

   _____

Answer the questions above and complete the *Point-of-Care Testing (POCT)* activity on the Student CD under Chapter 5 before you continue to the next section.

5-7 Urine Specimens

Urinalysis is a tool used to evaluate the substances found in urine. Urine tests can help determine the state of the human body if collected and analyzed properly. Because the urine test is a basic screening test, all abnormal signs should be followed up by a confirmation test (see Figure 5-12). A phlebotomist may be asked to perform a urine dipstick test. A complete urinalysis consists of three parts. The physical component has to do with the color, odor, and clarity of the urine. The chemical component consists of the following parts: protein, bilirubin, urobilinogen, ketones, pH, specific gravity, blood, leukocytes, nitrites, and glucose. The microscopic component consists of pouring urine into a centrifuge tube, then spinning it down to obtain the sediment. The sediment is used to make a slide to view under a microscope to check for various cells, bacteria, yeast, or other pathogens.

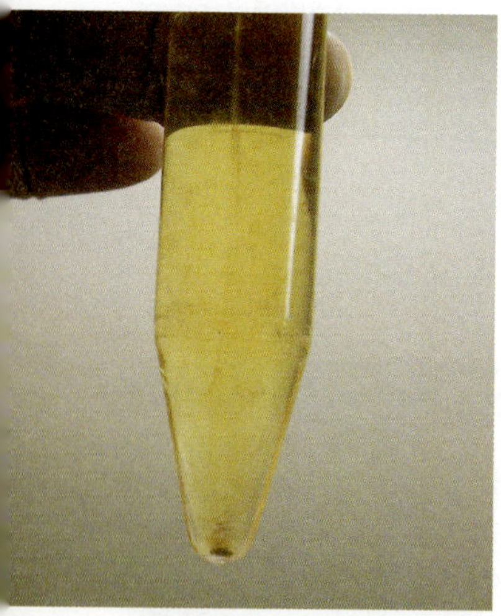

The best urine specimen for testing would be the first morning void, which is the most concentrated. Another type of specimen to collect, preferably in an outpatient setting, would be a clean-catch midstream specimen. Other urine specimen types would include random, timed, and 24-hour.

Sometimes you may need to obtain urine specimens for drug or alcohol testing. If so, you must establish a chain of custody. As discussed earlier in this chapter, this procedure requires you to fill out paperwork showing specific identification, who obtained and processed the specimen, the date, the location, and the signature of the patient documenting that the specimen in the container is the one that was obtained from the person identified on the label. The specimen must be placed in a specimen transfer bag that permanently seals the specimen bag until it is cut open

Figure 5-12 Once a urine specimen is centrifuged, the sediment in the bottom of the tube is analyzed by a microscope.

for analysis. The seal ensures that there has been no tampering with the contents of the bag before it reaches the lab for testing.

If the urine is not tested within one hour after it has been collected, it must be refrigerated. If urine is kept at room temperature for more than one hour it can alter the test results of the chemical and microscopic components.

Obtaining Urine Specimens

The phlebotomist, if working in a satellite office, may be required to collect a urine specimen from a patient; therefore, it is important to give specific information to the patient concerning the proper way to collect the specimen. If the patient is in the hospital a specimen can be obtained from the catheter bag, or the nurse may do a straight catheter to obtain a specimen that way. The directions for obtaining a clean-catch specimen are as follows:

- Female
  - Separate the skin folds (labia), take one antiseptic towelette and wipe from front to back down one side of the skin folds, and discard the towelette. Take a second towelette and wipe down the other side of the skin folds from front to back; discard the towelette. Take a third towelette and wipe down the middle of the labia front to back and discard the towelette.
  - Keeping the skin folds spread apart to avoid contamination, have the patient start to urinate into the toilet. Place the cup under the flow of urine. That's why it's called clean-catch midstream.
  - Once the patient is finished he or she should place the lid on the cup. Ideally the cup should be about three-fourths full.
  - Label the specimen (name, date of collection). Remember, your facility might require other identification on the specimen so check with your supervisor or procedure manual for further instructions.

- Male
  - Use an antiseptic towelette to clean the head of the penis. Take a second towelette and wipe across the head of the penis. If the patient is uncircumcised, retract the foreskin before cleaning the penis.
  - If uncircumcised keep foreskin retracted and tell the patient to urinate into the toilet. Place the cup under the stream as the patient urinates to collect a urine sample.
  - Once the patient is finished have the patient place the lid on the cup. Ideally the cup should be about three-fourths full.
  - Label the specimen (name, date of collection). Remember, your facility might require other identification on the specimen so check with your supervisor or procedure manual for further instructions.

Remember to label the specimen completely and properly and transport to the laboratory for immediate testing (see Figure 5-13).

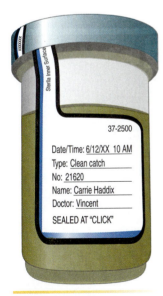

Figure 5-13 A urine specimen should include the patient's name, identification number, and/or birth date, and the date and time of collection, plus the method of collection.

Urine Specimen Testing

As a phlebotomist you will not be asked to perform a microscopic urinalysis; however, you may be required to perform a urine dipstick. A urine dipstick is one type of waived point-of-care test. It is done with a reagent strip. Reagents (on plastic strips) are chemicals that react with a particular substance in urine and change color in precise ways. These changes indicate the presence of that substance and the amount or concentration of the substance in the urine specimen. For example, when a reagent strip is used to test for ketones, the color on the strip, after it is allowed to react with the urine for the proper amount of time, will correspond to a specific concentration of ketone bodies. Alternately the test could be negative or no ketones present.

Reagent strips are used to test urine for a number of substances. In addition to ketones, these substances include nitrite, pH, blood, bilirubin, glucose, specific gravity, protein, and leukocytes.

There are numerous trade names for urine reagent strips, or dipsticks (for example, Multistix® and Chemstrip®). Not all reagents are reactive for the same chemicals. You must choose the appropriate strip according to the chemical test requested. All reagent strips are used once and discarded.

Follow the exact directions that come with the reagent strips to ensure accurate results. For quality assurance, take these basic precautions: Keep strips in tightly closed containers in a cool, dry area. Never remove them from the container until immediately before testing. Never touch the pads on the strip with your fingers or gloved hands. Examine strips for discoloration before use; discard discolored strips (see Figure 5-14). Check the expiration date on the bottle; do not use strips that have expired. Use strips within six months of opening the container. Every time you open a new supply of reagents, run control samples to check for proper operation. Write the date opened on the bottle. Although the process is essentially the same for all reagent strip tests, there are variations in time intervals before reading results. Some reagent strips are designed to test for several substances at once. (All time intervals start from time zero.)

Figure 5-14 Reagent strips are dipped into the urine specimen and then compared to colors on the reagent bottle to determine the results.

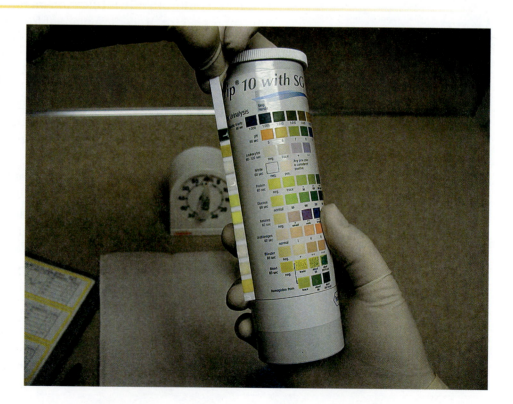

1. How soon should a urine specimen be tested if it is not refrigerated?

   _____

   _____

   _____

2. What is a reagent strip and how is it used?

   _____

   _____

   _____

   _____

Answer the questions above and complete the *Urine Specimen* activity on the Student CD under Chapter 5 before you continue to the next section.

5-8 Centrifuge Operation

Phlebotomists not only are required to draw patient specimens, but in many places of employment, they may also be expected to centrifuge blood and possibly urine samples. Specimen processing can be a separate section of a large laboratory, and for the phlebotomist, this presents an opportunity to aid in the testing procedure. Processing involves centrifuging (spinning down or separating the cells from the liquid portion of the blood) and **aliquoting** (dividing or separating specimens into separate containers) patient samples. For most laboratory tests that require serum or plasma, it is recommended that specimens be separated within two hours of collection or less. If samples were not centrifuged or aliquoted within two hours, the laboratory test results could be altered. If the red blood cells were left in contact with the serum or plasma, glucose would be decreased and potassium can significantly increase because cells use glucose to keep themselves alive and nourished. This is known as glycolysis. Potassium and glucose blood tests are most affected, as are coagulation studies, when the blood is allowed to sit for longer than two hours.

Centrifuges come in many different styles: refrigerated, floor models, and tabletop models. The speed of rotation (revolutions per minute, or rpm) and the radius of the rotor head determine the relative centrifugal force (RCF) of a centrifuge. The relative centrifugal force is expressed as gravity (g). Most laboratory specimens are centrifuged at 750 to 1000 g for 15 minutes.

Centrifuges are designed to spin blood specimens down, separating the cells from the liquid portion. Different size tubes can be spun in the same centrifuge at the same time. Be sure to place tubes of equal size and volume directly across from each other (see Figure 5-15). Also, make sure that the levels of sample are the same so that the centrifuge will be balanced. If you do not have an even number of blood tubes to spin, you can balance the centrifuge with a similar tube filled with water or saline.

After the lid has been securely closed, turn the centrifuge on for 15 minutes or the designated time. Wait until the centrifuge has reached its running

Figure 5-15 Place tubes of equal size and volume directly across from each other so the centrifuge is balanced.

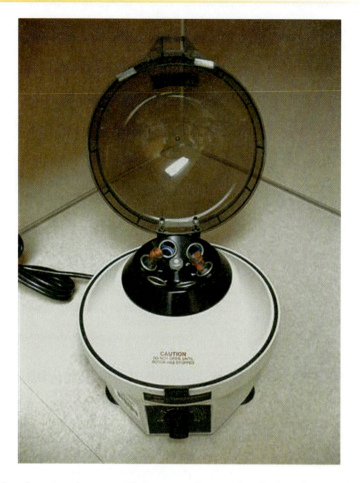

speed before leaving the area. If the centrifuge is loaded with samples that are not balanced, the centrifuge will vibrate and make noise. If you are nearby, you can turn off the centrifuge before the unbalanced samples are broken. The centrifuge must be calibrated on a regular schedule with a tachometer to ensure proper centrifugation.

Improper use of a centrifuge can be dangerous to the user and can ruin laboratory specimens. If a tube is broken, the cup containing the broken tube must be completely emptied into a sharps container and disinfected. Never open a centrifuge lid until the rotor has come to a complete stop. There could be a glass tube that might have shattered during the centrifuge process. If you open the lid before it stops, you could run the risk of being injured by the flying glass or debris.

The prevention of aerosols (a mist that travels in the air) escaping when stoppers are removed or in uncovered tubes that are centrifuged is a major concern of laboratory personnel. Aerosols can contain viruses and would endanger a person if inhaled. Several shields are available for this purpose and, when used properly, they greatly reduce the exposure to aerosols. The shields or splashguards are designed as a barrier between the person and the aerosol created by removing a tube top.

Careful attention to detail is imperative when aliquoting patient specimens. Mixing up patient samples is one of the greatest concerns of all laboratory workers. Before you begin to aliquot a sample, make sure the transfer tube is properly labeled by comparing it to the label on the specimen tube that was used for collection.

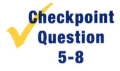
1. What tests would be affected the most if not centrifuged at the appropriate time?

_____

_____

_____

_____

_____

 Answer the question above and complete the *Centrifuge Operation* activity on the Student CD under Chapter 5 before you continue to the next section.

Chapter Summary

- Specimens may require special handling or collection in order to be accurate. Pre-analytical errors can occur before, during, and after collection when these procedures are not followed exactly.

- Blood cultures must be drawn under strict aseptic technique to prevent false positives. Every set of cultures has one aerobic and one anaerobic specimen, and more than one set of cultures are frequently taken to ensure against false negatives.

- When using a Unopette®, collect the specimen with the pipette. Place a gloved finger over the reservoir and mix by inversion, then carefully squeeze the reservoir to mix the specimen.

- To perform a microhematocrit, you must obtain blood in a capillary tube and spin in a microhematocrit centrifuge. The cells separate from the plasma in the tube and the tube is compared to a scale on the machine or portable scale to determine the patient's hematocrit.

- Peripheral blood smears require a drop of blood on a slide that is spread across the slide using a spreader slide. When complete, the smear is a thin tongue or bullet shape, does not go to the edge of the slide, and is feathered.

- Point-of-care tests are obtained and tested immediately at the point of care or near the patient. CLIA waived tests are performed in a certified laboratory, are FDA approved, and pose a minimal risk of harm to the patient. Strict regulations including frequent calibration of test machines is mandated.

- A urine specimen can be collected from a catheter or from a patient using the clean-catch method. When dipped in urine, the reagent strip changes color to indicate the presence and/or concentration of a substance in a urine specimen.

- When using a centrifuge make sure the load is balanced. If it makes noise turn it off immediately to prevent breakage. Wait until the centrifuge has stopped completely before opening and use a shield or mask, as required, when opening.

Chapter Review

Multiple Choice

Circle the best response for each of the following questions.

1. Anaerobic means:
   a. Air loving
   b. Nothing to eat
   c. Room air
   d. Without air

2. The aseptic collection of blood cultures requires that the skin be cleaned with:
   a. Soap and water
   b. 70% alcohol and then 95% alcohol
   c. 70%–95% alcohol and then 2% iodine
   d. 95% alcohol only

3. Which of the following procedures would help diagnose an infection caused by *Mycoplasma pneumoniae?*
   a. Blood cultures
   b. Blood smear
   c. Bleeding time
   d. Cold agglutinins

4. Which of the following is true concerning bleeding time?
   a. The test is performed to assess platelet function.
   b. A stopwatch is started at the same time that the puncture is made.
   c. You touch only the drop of blood, not the skin, with the filter paper.
   d. All of the above

5. When making a blood smear, the angle used to make the smear is:
   a. 10 degrees
   b. 20 degrees
   c. 30 degrees
   d. 45 degrees

6. When aliquoting specimens a shield or splashguard is used to protect the phlebotomist from:
   a. Aerosols
   b. Normal flora
   c. Bacteremia
   d. Septicemia

7. Which of the following anticoagulants is found in a red-tipped microhematocrit tube?
   a. Sodium heparin
   b. Ammonium oxalate
   c. EDTA
   d. Sodium citrate

8. Which statement describes proper centrifuge operation?
   a. Centrifuge specimens within five minutes of collection.
   b. Balance specimens by placing tubes of equal size and volume opposite each other.
   c. Never centrifuge plasma specimens with serum specimens.
   d. Remove tops from tubes before centrifuging.

9. Which of the following tests requires an arterial specimen?
   a. Ammonia
   b. Blood culture
   c. Blood gases
   d. Microhematocrit

10. What tests may be affected most if the patient is not fasting?
    a. CBC and prothrombin
    b. Glucose and triglycerides
    c. Blood culture and bleeding time
    d. Blood gases and microhematocrit

11. _____ are designed to spin blood specimens down, separating the cells from the liquid portion.
    a. Colter machines
    b. Holter monitors
    c. Centrifuges
    d. None of the above

12. The purpose of _____ is to reduce the turnaround time for blood test results. Some of the types of tests are glucose, hemoglobin, sodium, potassium, chloride, and cholesterol, just to name a few.
    a. Waived testing
    b. Reference lab testing
    c. Point-of-care testing
    d. None of the above

13. The volume of blood collected for a blood culture is critical. Each manufacturer of blood culture bottles or tubes has determined the optimum amount of blood sample needed. Usually _____ to _____ millimeters for each bottle or tube is sufficient.
    a. 1 to 6
    b. 8 to 10
    c. 3 to 8
    d. None of the above

14. The primary purpose of cleansing the venipuncture site is to:
    a. Reduce the number of normal flora at the selected puncture site
    b. Increase the site by which you draw blood
    c. Create a barrier for the microbes
    d. None of the above

15. Urine specimens are sometimes tested using a:
  a. Pipette
  b. Reagent strip
  c. Unopette®
  d. Capillary tube

True or False

Write T or F in the blank to indicate whether you think the statement is true or false. Correct any false statements to make them true.

_____ **16.** It is important to obtain a blood culture specimen from two different locations.

_____ **17.** Testing for cold agglutinins is done for patients suspected of having conditions such as atypical pneumonia.

_____ **18.** The most common type of POCT is potassium.

_____ **19.** If urine is kept at room temperature for more than two hours it can alter the test results of the chemical and microscopic components.

_____ **20.** The lid on the centrifuge machine should be properly closed during the centrifuging process.

Matching

Match each key term with the correct definition by writing the appropriate letter in the space provided.

_____ **21.** waived test

_____ **22.** differential

_____ **23.** chain of custody

_____ **24.** septicemia

_____ **25.** cold agglutinin

_____ **26.** bacteremia

_____ **27.** Unopette®

_____ **28.** false positive

_____ **29.** false negative

_____ **30.** pre-analytical error

a. Identifying and securing a specimen

b. Nonspecific autoantibody present with *Mycoplasma pneumoniae*

c. Suggests an abnormality erroneously

d. Occurs before a specimen is analyzed

e. Collection system designed for hematology tests that uses diluted whole blood

f. Microscopic examination of a stained monolayer blood smear

g. Presence of microorganisms in the blood usually with symptoms

h. Presence of bacteria in the blood

i. Must be approved by the FDA

j. Suggests no abnormality erroneously

What Should You Do?

Use your critical thinking skills to respond to the following situations.

31. You are working in the processing area of the laboratory and notice that a specimen you were just given was drawn over two days ago. This is the same blood sample for which a doctor just called for the results. He was upset and wanted the results immediately. What would you do?

   _____

   _____

   _____

   _____

32. You have finished labeling all of Mrs. Diaz's blood tubes when you notice that one sample was to be put on ice immediately. You have been talking to Mrs. Diaz for the last ten minutes. What would you do?

   _____

   _____

   _____

   _____

33. You have orders to obtain blood cultures × 2. You have finished the procedure, but you can't remember if you did the initial cleansing of the skin. What would be your reaction as a phlebotomist?

   _____

   _____

   _____

   _____

Get Connected *Internet Activity*

Visit the McGraw-Hill Higher Education Online Learning Center *Phlebotomy for Health Care Personnel* Website at **www.mhhe.com/healthcareskills** to complete the following activity.

1. Visit the Centers for Disease Control and Prevention Division of Laboratory Systems, and learn more about pre-analytical errors and how they can be avoided. From your research, discover the six factors that influence the quality of the specimen and prevent pre-analytical errors.

Using the Student CD

Now that you have completed the material in the chapter text, return to the Student CD and complete any chapter activities you have not yet done. Practice your terminology with the "Key Term Concentration" game. Review the chapter material with the "Spin the Wheel" game. Take the final chapter test and complete the troubleshooting question. E-mail or print your results to document your proficiency for this chapter.

6 Special Phlebotomy Procedures

Learning Outcomes

Upon completion of this chapter, you should be able to:

- Discuss why specimen collections should be drawn at specified times.
- Name two tests that require fasting.
- Describe various types of glucose tests.
- Explain the purpose of bleeding time.
- Identify standard protocol and procedure for blood donation.
- Compare and contrast blood donations, therapeutic phlebotomy, and autologous donation.
- Discuss the precautions associated with blood alcohol testing.
- Differentiate between forensic and toxicology specimens.
- Explain the reasons for therapeutic drug monitoring.
- List other sites for blood specimen collection.

Key Terms

analyte	hemochromatosis
assay	keloid
bleeding time	lipemic
cannula	Platelet Function Assay (PFA)
diabetes mellitus	polycythemia
disinfectant	reference values
diurnal variation	sphygmomanometer
gestational diabetes	therapeutic drug monitoring
glycolysis	therapeutic medication

6-1 Introduction

The phlebotomist must be equipped with knowledge of special laboratory tests. Special tests include timed specimens, glucose tolerance testing, therapeutic phlebotomy collections, bleeding time, blood alcohol, toxicology, chain-of-custody specimens, and therapeutic monitoring of drug levels. Some of these tests require additional preparation and some tests require extra skills. Licensed practitioners depend on the phlebotomist to know the special requirements and adhere to them. Following these special procedures will directly impact the quality of patient care. Patients can affect laboratory results by exercising, eating, fasting, lying down, standing up, being stressed, smoking, or drinking alcohol. Table 6-1 is a list of some laboratory tests that can be affected by different patient behaviors. Phlebotomists are also given the opportunity to educate patients about the laboratory and the importance of following the physician's directions.

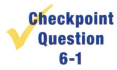

Checkpoint Question 6-1

1. Name at least four patient behaviors that can affect test results.

_____

_____

_____

_____

_____

6-2 Timed Specimens

Laboratory requisitions will frequently note the time a blood sample should be drawn. Some reasons for specimens to be drawn at a specified time include **therapeutic medication** blood levels; monitoring changes in a patient's condition, such as cardiac enzymes for a heart patient; measuring the body's ability to metabolize a certain substance; or even measuring **analytes** (substances undergoing analysis) that exhibit diurnal variation. **Diurnal variation** is the variation of analyte levels during different times throughout the day. Certain laboratory tests require special patient preparation and timing of the sample to be collected. Laboratory tests that are collected at a specified time include peak and trough medication levels for drug monitoring, glucose tolerance tests (GTTs), iron levels, hormone **assays** (lab analyses), cortisol levels, and cardiac enzymes. The phlebotomist must understand why preparation of the patient before the collection and timing of the collection can be critical to a patient's care and well-being.

Fasting

The expected or **reference values** that are published for many laboratory tests are determined using patient specimens from volunteers who are considered normal or in good health. These volunteers are also asked to be fasting (abstaining from food) and in a basal state (absence of exercise). Fasting and basal state specimens are usually drawn first thing in the morning,

TABLE 6-1 Some Patient Variables That Affect Laboratory Tests

Variables	Tests Affected
Nonfasting	Glucose Triglycerides
Stress	Adrenal hormones Fatty acids Lactate White blood cells
Posture	Albumin Bilirubin Calcium Enzymes Lipids Total protein Red blood cells White blood cells
Exercise	Aldolase Creatinine Fatty acids Lactate Sex hormones AST CK LD White blood cells
Diurnal variations	Cortisol Serum iron White blood cells
Alcohol	Lactate Triglycerides Uric acid GGT HDL
Tobacco	Cathecholamines Cortisol Hemoglobin White blood cells

following hours of sleep and little activity. This makes the fasting period less stressful for the patient. Fasting is the most common timed specimen request. Patients are asked to abstain from food and beverages (except water) for 8 to 12 hours before the venipuncture and to avoid all strenuous activities prior to the blood test.

Not all laboratory tests require fasting; however, some chemistry analyses require that a patient fast for 12 hours prior to venipuncture. The tests most affected by not fasting are glucose and triglycerides. If blood is drawn shortly after a meal, the serum may appear cloudy or **lipemic**

Figure 6-1 The lipemic serum sample on the right is very milky compared to the normal (clear) serum.

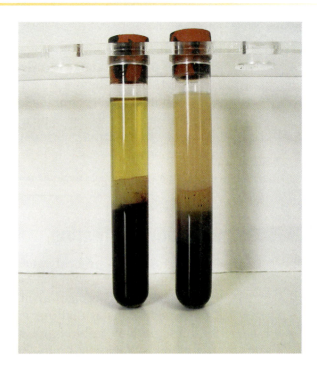

(see Figure 6-1). Lipemia is due to the large amount of fatty compounds in blood after a meal, and it will interfere with many laboratory tests. Severely lipemic specimens have an appearance similar to milk instead of the normal serum appearance of clear yellow fluid. Many laboratory tests can be drawn at any time throughout the day because eating or exercise has little affect on the results.

Checkpoint Questions 6-2

1. How long are patients required to fast before certain blood tests?

_____

_____

_____

_____

2. What tests are most affected by non-fasting?

_____

_____

_____

_____

_____

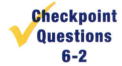

Answer the questions above and complete the *Timed Specimens* activity on the Student CD under Chapter 6 before you continue to the next section.

Fasting

It is important for the licensed practitioner, nurse, or laboratory staff to inform patients about fasting. Fasting means nothing to eat or drink for 8 to 12 hours before blood is to be collected. However, water is allowed and even encouraged. Abstaining from water can result in dehydration, which can cause erroneous laboratory results. Written laboratory instructions with detailed explanations should be provided to all patients.

6-3 Glucose Testing

Glucose testing is probably the most frequently ordered laboratory test. Glucose levels aid the physician in diagnosing **diabetes mellitus,** gestational diabetes, hyperinsulinism, and other related glucose abnormalities. If untreated, diabetes mellitus can lead to many complications including blindness, kidney failure, and amputation resulting from problems with circulation in the lower limbs. An increase in blood glucose is an indicator of this disease; however, the patient's fasting glucose level may be within normal limits. A physician may thus order a glucose tolerance test, insulin level, or a series of tests to determine the patient's medical problem.

A two-hour postprandial glucose test is sometimes ordered. Glucose levels obtained two hours after a meal can be elevated in diabetic patients but are generally within normal range for most of the population. Ideally, in two hours the glucose level will have returned to normal. Correct timing is important because if collected too early, the glucose level may still be elevated and may lead to misinterpretation of the test results by the physician.

Glucose Tolerance Test (GTT)

A glucose tolerance test measures a patient's ability to metabolize a large oral dose of glucose. Although used less commonly, the classic oral glucose tolerance test measures blood glucose levels five times over a period of three hours. Some physicians simply get a baseline blood sample followed by a sample two hours after drinking the glucose solution. A glucose challenge screening test is frequently done to test for **gestational diabetes.** Gestational diabetes is elevated blood sugar that occurs during pregnancy. During a glucose challenge test the patient is given oral glucose and a blood sample is drawn one hour later. If this test is positive, then a complete GTT is done. See Table 6-2 for types of glucose tests.

To begin, fasting blood and urine specimens are collected. The patient's blood glucose level is determined, and if the blood glucose level is over 200 mg/dL, no further testing is required. It is unsafe to give a patient with elevated blood sugar additional glucose. It could cause nausea or extremely elevated blood sugar. If the glucose level is less than 200 mg/dL, the GTT should be continued.

A loading dose of glucose (a special drink purchased by laboratories containing a known amount of dissolved glucose) is given to the patient to

TABLE 6-2 Glucose Tests

Name	Purpose	Test and Timing
Fasting blood sugar (FBS)	To identify risk of diabetes	Single blood sample after no intake of food or drink for 8 to 12 hours
2-hour postprandial blood sugar (2-hour PP)	To identify risk of diabetes	Taken exactly two hours after a meal; used less frequently because of inconsistent results
Random blood sugar (RBS)	To identify risk of diabetes or hypoglycemia	Taken randomly throughout day; a wide variety of results indicates possible problem
2- or 3-hour oral glucose tolerance test (OGTT)	To diagnose gestational diabetes, diabetes mellitus, hypothalamic obesity, and reactive hypoglycemia	Fasting blood sugar, 30 minutes, 1 hour, 2 hours, and 3 hours after oral glucose
Glucose challenge screening test	To identify risk of gestational diabetes (1 hour) or polycystic ovary syndrome (2 hour)	Blood sample 1 hour or 2 hours after oral glucose
Intravenous glucose tolerance test (IVGTT)	To evaluate insulin secretion in prediabetics	Blood samples are taken after glucose is administered through an IV or directly into the bloodstream

drink. If the GTT is to be performed on a child, follow the instructions on the side of the bottle. Children are typically given a certain number of ounces of glucose solution according to their weight.

The phlebotomist must ensure that all of the glucose solution is swallowed within five minutes and that no vomiting has occurred. Specimens are usually drawn in gray-topped tubes that contain a substance to prevent the breakdown of glucose, which helps ensure accurate results.

At each of these times a urine sample is also collected. Care should be taken to label each sample (blood and urine) with both the time collected and the time interval (for example, 30 minutes, 1 hour, 2 hours, or 3 hours). Patients should not leave the facility during the test, and no food, alcohol, smoking, or gum chewing is allowed for the duration of the tolerance test. The patient is allowed to consume water, however. All specimens should be centrifuged soon after the sample has clotted to prevent **glycolysis** (the breaking down of glucose into an acid). Both urine and serum glucose levels should be run shortly after collection, not as part of the routine laboratory specimens. The laboratory sends the ordering physician the results of the GTT, which assists the physician in determining the presence and type of diabetes as well as the appropriate treatment.

Glucose Tolerance Test

Patients who arrive for a glucose tolerance test must be fasting, and then are given a large dose of glucose (sugar). This makes them prone to syncope (fainting). It is imperative that the phlebotomist go out to the waiting area to meet patients and walk with them back to the lab. The phlebotomist should not just call a patient's name and wait for him or her to come to the drawing area. The phlebotomist should also escort patients back to the waiting area after the draw, and make sure they are settled and feeling stable. The phlebotomist should be ready to steady the patient if needed, and to react appropriately should the patient pass out. Patients can fall and hurt themselves, putting the phlebotomist at risk for a lawsuit. It is also recommended to have a large container close by in case the patient becomes nauseated and throws up. Due to the high load of glucose on an empty stomach, this is a very common occurrence. Additionally, patients should be monitored to assure they do not "sneak a snack" or drink during the testing time, which could interfere with the results.

Checkpoint Questions 6-3

1. Why is it necessary to monitor the patient carefully during a glucose tolerance test?

_____

_____

_____

_____

2. A pregnant patient is at risk for gestational diabetes. What test would be done first?

_____

_____

_____

_____

Answer the questions above and complete the *Glucose Testing* activity on the Student CD under Chapter 6 before you continue to the next section.

6-4 Bleeding Time and Platelet Function

Bleeding time is the time it takes a standardized skin wound to stop bleeding. The bleeding time test measures the ability of the platelets to stop bleeding after an injury. The bleeding time test helps assess the ability of platelets to function during a bleeding episode. The device used to perform a bleeding time produces a standard incision 5 mm long and 1 mm deep when placed firmly on the patient's forearm.

Normal bleeding time is 2.5 to 9.5 minutes. Many situations can cause a prolonged bleeding time. These include platelet dysfunction, decreased platelet number, fibrinogen disorders, and medications that hinder platelet functions. Medications that interfere with platelet function include aspirin, aspirin-containing medications, nonsteroidal anti-inflammatory agents, and antihistamines.

The **Platelet Function Assay (PFA)** test has proven to be an acceptable test to determine platelet adhesion and aggregation (primary hemostasis). The PFA is replacing the bleeding time test because the bleeding time test has proven to be very insensitive to patients who use aspirin or nonsteroidal anti-inflammatory agents. (The use of these medications can change the results.) In addition, the PFA test is less invasive, requiring a simple venipuncture. When performing a PFA test, you will need to collect two light blue-topped citrate tubes. These tubes should not be refrigerated and must be delivered to the laboratory within one hour of collection.

Performing the Bleeding Time Procedure

Place the patient's arm on a steady support with the palm facing up. Select a site for the bleeding time procedure midway down the forearm; usually the ventral side of the arm is used. The puncture should be about 2 cm distal to the antecubital fossa. Select a site that is free of exposed veins, rashes, scars, and bruises. Shave the site if the patient has a notable amount of hair. Place the **sphygmomanometer** (blood pressure cuff) on the patient's upper arm instead of a tourniquet.

Patient Education & Communication

Keloids

Before performing a bleeding time test, the phlebotomist must inform the patient of the possibility of a scar as a result of the procedure. Patients who scar easily or tend to form **keloids** (enlarged scars due to excessive collagen formation) should be warned of the scarring possibility. Indicate on the laboratory requisition that the patient was informed of the potential for scarring.

Cleanse the site with an alcohol prep pad and allow the area to air dry. Remove the bleeding time device from the packaging and remove the safety clip from the device. Be careful not to contaminate the device before use. Inflate the sphygmomanometer to 40 mmHg. Make sure the pressure on the sphygmomanometer stays at 40 mmHg for the duration of the bleeding time procedure to maintain this standard, consistent amount of pressure.

Rest the bleeding time device on the patient's forearm parallel to the antecubital crease (i.e., across the arm). Apply minimal but firm pressure. Both ends of the device should just touch the skin. Simultaneously push the trigger, which will create a slice in the skin, and start the stopwatch (see Figure 6-2). The phlebotomist begins timing from the start (puncture) of the test and continues until the bleeding has completely stopped. Immediately after making the incision, remove the device and properly dispose of it into a sharps container. After 30 seconds wick the flow of blood using filter paper. Do not touch the filter paper directly to the incision site; this will cause the

Figure 6-2 Apply a bleeding time instrument and make the bleeding time incision.

Figure 6-3 Wick the blood using filter paper.

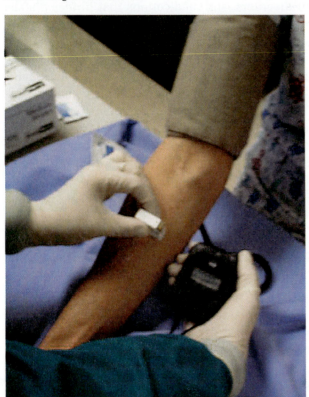

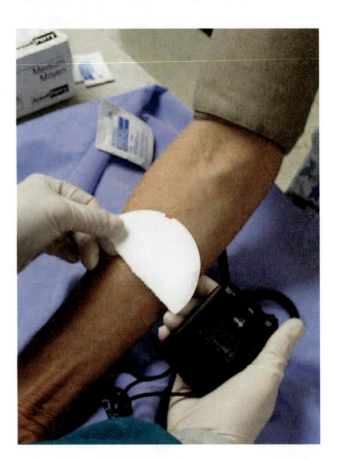

forming clot to break apart. Wick the incision every 30 seconds until the flow stops (see Figure 6-3). Stop the stopwatch. If the bleeding continues longer than 15 minutes, stop the procedure, apply pressure, and record the bleeding time as greater than 15 minutes.

Remove the sphygmomanometer and carefully clean around the incision area. Apply a bandage (a butterfly bandage if available) across the incision area. Try to squeeze or pull the two sides of the incision together while applying the butterfly bandage. The butterfly bandage should be left in place for 24 hours. Bleeding times are reported to the nearest 30 seconds. You can simply look at the stopwatch to determine the bleeding time results.

Troubleshooting Notify the Physician

A phlebotomist must never instruct a patient not to take a medication. If a laboratory result is dependent on a patient taking or not taking a certain medication the physician should be notified. For example, if a patient has a prolonged bleeding time and has taken one of the medicines known to inhibit platelet function, the ordering physician should be notified. It is up to the licensed practitioner to reorder the procedure and to inform the patient to stop the medicine before the test is repeated.

Question: Name three medications that inhibit platelet function and about which the physician should be informed if a patient is having a bleeding time test.

_____

_____

_____

_____

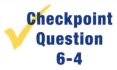
Checkpoint Question 6-4

1. Why is the PFA test replacing the bleeding time test?

_____

_____

_____

_____

 Answer the question above and complete the _Bleeding Time and Platelet Function_ activity on the Student CD under Chapter 6 before you continue to the next section.

6-5 Therapeutic Collection and Blood Donation

Therapeutic phlebotomy and blood donation both require the intentional collection of a large volume of blood. Therapeutic phlebotomies are performed for many medical reasons, usually to reduce stress on the body systems due to overproduction of iron or red blood cells or an abnormal storage mechanism of iron. Therapeutic phlebotomy and blood donation are performed the same: A vein is accessed and one unit of blood is removed. Patients undergoing therapeutic phlebotomy are not usually as healthy as normal blood donors, so they require closer monitoring (see Figure 6-4). Usually 500 mL are taken during one treatment. The blood would not be suitable for a blood transfusion and is therefore discarded.

Therapeutic Collections

Therapeutic phlebotomy is most commonly used as a method of treatment for polycythemia. **Polycythemia** is a disease that causes an overproduction or abnormal increase in the number of red blood cells. An increased number of red blood cells can be detrimental to a patient's overall health. The increase in red blood cells puts the heart and other organs under a tremendous amount of strain in trying to circulate this abnormally high number of cells.

Another reason a physician would order a therapeutic phlebotomy would be for treatment of hemochromatosis. **Hemochromatosis** is a disease in which the body stores iron in abnormal amounts. The patient with

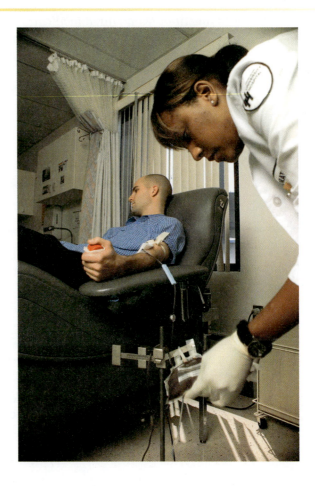

hemochromatosis has an overabundance of iron throughout his or her body. This iron overload can cause many serious health problems, and measures need to be taken to reduce the iron level. Therapeutic phlebotomy is the most common treatment for this condition.

Blood Donation

Blood donations are performed by a phlebotomist. Each donor unit can yield the following life-saving products:

- Red blood cells
- Plasma
- Platelets
- Blood clotting factors
- Blood typing reagents
- Proteins and immunoglobins

Blood products are separated into components at a donor facility. Blood donor vans travel to many remote locations, but the process of making components is usually performed at the donor laboratory or facility. The American Red Cross is one such facility. All blood products require meticulous labeling so that each unit can easily be traced back to the blood donor.

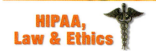

Blood Collection

Blood is considered a regulated drug according to the U.S. Food and Drug Administration (FDA). For this reason significant training is required for a phlebotomist to be deemed competent to collect blood for future transfusions. In addition to accurate identification, the patient must be interviewed and screened carefully. Additionally, the patient may be required to have a mini physical examination. As a phlebotomist, you must obtain the proper training and follow the guidelines set forth by the facility where you are employed before collecting blood for further transfusion.

Unlike for therapeutic phlebotomy, which is done to improve the patient's health status by removing blood, blood donation candidates must meet the requirements for blood donation. First, individuals must be interviewed to determine appropriate age, weight, and overall health status. Blood donors must weigh at least 110 pounds and be between 17 and 66 years of age. Written parental consent is required for minors. A hematocrit or hemoglobin should be of sufficient levels to ensure the safety of the donor. Health status and permission for the blood to be used by the blood bank is obtained during the brief physical examination and complete health history. Part of the history screening process includes questions regarding recent travel out of the country and sexual activity. Some patients have been surprised at the depth of questioning regarding their sexual activity, and they need to be assured that it is to help screen for sexually transmitted diseases (STDs) and human immunodeficiency virus (HIV).

Patients need to be made aware of the need to ensure a safe blood supply. Pressure to donate through work, school, and church can put these patients in an awkward position when answering questions. It may be difficult for some people to admit to others that they may have put themselves at risk due to some past experiences. It is very important to let them know that they will have another opportunity to alert the staff to possible contamination without others being made aware of it.

Once the initial screenings are completed, donors are placed in a comfortable sitting or reclining position. Comfort is important, since the procedure takes approximately seven minutes to collect one donor unit of 450 to 500 milliliters. The preferred site of venipuncture is from a large antecubital vein. A two-step skin cleansing process, similar to the process for blood culture collection, is followed. Blood units are collected in a sterile, closed collection system consisting of the blood collection bag to collect the blood, tubing, and a 16-gauge needle. Once the vein is accessed, blood flows via gravity into the collection bag, which is placed lower than the donor's arm. An anticoagulant, citrate phosphate dextrose (CPD-A1) in solution, is present in the blood collection bag. During the collection process, the phlebotomist may place the bag on a mixing unit next to the patient. The mixing agitates the contents, which ensures that the blood is being mixed properly with the anticoagulant. In some facilities the phlebotomist performs manual mixing by gently manipulating the bag as the blood flows into it. This sterile, closed blood collection unit is to be used only once. If for some reason the bag does not fill with blood, the needle and the blood collection bag must be discarded. If this occurs, the entire process will have to be repeated using another blood donor collection setup. This is done to maintain the sterility of the donor unit.

As mentioned in Chapter 2, individuals can donate blood for their future use. This is referred to as autologous blood donation (see Figure 6-5). The blood can be placed on reserve for the individual to use within a certain amount of time. If the patient is donating blood prior to a surgical procedure, certain prerequisites must be met. First, the patient must have a written order from a physician and be capable of regenerating red blood cells. In other words, the patient must be in good enough health to replace the blood donation. In addition, the individual's hemoglobin must be at least 11 grams, and the surgical procedure must be scheduled for more than 72 hours from the time of autologous donation. Autologous donations continue to gain popularity, primarily because of the increased concern about transmission of bloodborne pathogens such as HIV.

During and following any type of blood donation, patients must be monitored for potential side effects such as dizziness and nausea. If dizziness occurs, keep the donor in a reclining position, preferably with the head lower than the heart. Do not allow the donor to stand or walk, for this may lead to injury as a result of fainting or falling. After the donation, a small snack and fruit juice usually prevent these common side effects from occurring. The blood glucose level of the donor could be lower than normal because of the donation of a unit of blood. The snack

Figure 6-5 Donated blood can be processed into a number of products. A patient can donate blood for his or her own future use. This is known as an autologous blood donation.

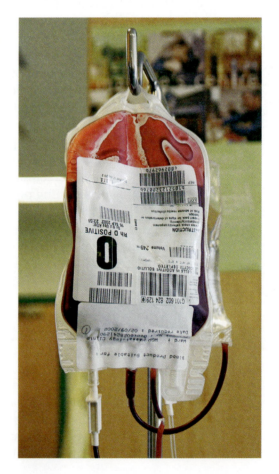

and fruit juice help increase the glucose level quickly before the patient leaves the area.

At the end of the donation procedure, the patient will be given a card with two bar code labels. Over the bar codes is a statement reiterating the importance of protecting the health of the future recipient, and asking if the patient considers his or her blood safe for transfusion. There is a YES or NO above each sticker. The patient is given the card, told to read it, and peel off one of the stickers and place it on the unit. The phlebotomist is to turn his or her back to the patient to allow for privacy. Then the phlebotomist should instruct the patient to fold the card after peeling off the sticker.

Patients may then dispose of the card so that no one else in the room can see which option they chose. This gives them one last chance to help ensure they will not put others at risk by using the blood donated. It can often take a while for someone to test positive for several pathogens, and by this method, the patient can make a safe choice, depending on current information available only to them.

✓ **Checkpoint Questions 6-5**

1. What type of blood collection is done for treatment of a disease? For use by a patient in the future?

_____

_____

_____

_____

_____

2. Why is it necessary to inform patients of the need for a safe blood supply?

_____

_____

_____

_____

_____

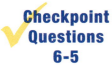

Answer the questions above and complete the *Blood Donation and Therapeutic Collection* activity on the Student CD under Chapter 6 before you continue to the next section.

6-6 Blood Alcohol, Toxicology, and Forensic Specimens

Certain special phlebotomy procedures require extra considerations regarding the patient, collection, and handling of the specimen. The special procedures discussed in this section include blood alcohol testing, toxicology, and forensic specimens.

Blood Alcohol Testing

Laboratory personnel determine blood alcohol levels. The police may request a blood alcohol level because of a possible DUI (driving under the influence). Before the test can be performed the patient must consent to having the test done. The patient can refuse to have the test done. If the phlebotomist attempts to collect a specimen for the test without written consent from the patient or a court order given, the phlebotomist can be found guilty of assault and battery, and the test will not be admissible in court. An employer may request a blood alcohol level because an employee smells or acts intoxicated. A phlebotomist performs the collection of the specimen for the blood alcohol. Care must be taken when collecting a blood alcohol specimen because these specimens are often needed for legal reasons, especially if the chain-of-custody routine is followed. The collection procedure is the same as routine venipuncture with the noted exception of the cleaning agent. An alcohol prep pad must *not* be used because it could cause a falsely elevated blood alcohol result. The venipuncture site must be cleaned with a **disinfectant** (solution containing an agent intended to kill microorganisms) other than alcohol, such as green surgical soap or hydrogen peroxide. Do not use iodine swabs because they also contain alcohol.

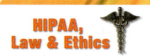

HIPAA, Law & Ethics

Legal Blood Alcohol Specimens

It is critical for the phlebotomist to understand that the patient has the right to refuse a blood alcohol specimen unless that right has been legally removed by an appropriate legal action. If it is being required due to an accident or where possible litigation may be involved, there must be a legal document, signed by the proper authorities, authorizing the draw. It is up to the phlebotomist to determine this is done before the draw. If not, the phlebotomist can be sued for assault and battery. If it is being ordered for possible litigation, a chain-of-custody form must also be filled out, and the top of the tube sealed with a tamper-proof label or wax.

Toxicology Specimens

Toxicology is the scientific study of poisons, drugs, or medications. Toxicologists are people who study the detection of poisons, the action of poisons on the human body, and the treatment of the medical conditions that poisons can cause. For toxicology specimens it is critical to follow your laboratory's protocol for collection, type of specimen, and equipment used in the collection process. Oil or bacteria from hands, glass, or plastic materials will contaminate or even react with some of the analytes.

Forensic Specimens

Forensic specimens usually involve testing specimens involved in legal cases. Forensic and legal specimens must follow a special chain-of-custody procedure. As discussed in Chapter 5, chain of custody requires

TABLE 6-3 Samples Collected for Forensic Purposes

- Blood
- Bones
- Hair
- Nails
- Saliva
- Skin
- Sperm
- Sweat
- Teeth
- Mud
- Vegetation

documentation that the specimen is accounted for at all times. The chain-of-custody procedure dictates that each person who handles the specimen must sign and date the legal document. The document indicates the name of the person from whom the specimen was received, the person to whom the specimen was given, and the length of time each person had the specimen. The specimen must be kept in a locked container and/or the tube is sealed with a tamper-proof label or wax at all times to prevent unauthorized personnel from tampering with the sample. The chain of custody gives accountability of the specimen from the time of collection to the final disposition of the specimen and guarantees the integrity of the specimen in a court of law.

The types of specimens collected listed in Table 6-3 are obtained and commonly used for forensic purposes. The primary aim of a forensic specimen is to collect evidence that may help prove or disprove a link between an individual and/or between individuals and objects or places. Some general guidelines should be followed when collecting forensic specimens.

- Avoid contamination by wearing gloves at all times.
- Collect the specimen as soon as possible.
- Ensure the specimen is packed, stored, and transported correctly. In general, fluids are refrigerated and other specimens are kept dry and at room temperature.
- Label each specimen with the patient's name, date of birth, the name of the person collecting the specimen, the type of specimen, and the date and time of the collection.
- Make sure the specimen is packed securely and is tamper-proof. Only authorized people should touch the specimen.
- Record all handling of the specimen, most commonly on a chain-of-custody form.

Most importantly, check the specific guidelines at your place of employment. In some cases you will use a special evidence kit (see Figure 6-6). Additionally, you should know the specific procedure and whether you have had the proper training to collect such specimens.

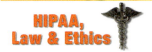

HIPAA, Law & Ethics

Following Protocols

It is the responsibility of the phlebotomist to ensure that all collection protocols are followed. If you collect a blood alcohol level you must take extra care that the site is cleaned with a non-alcohol cleanser. A contaminated or false positive result could cause the police officer to lose the court case, or a person to lose his job or even go to jail. Therefore the phlebotomist needs to be especially diligent in following all established collection protocols. A phlebotomist involved in collecting a blood alcohol specimen for legal reasons can be summoned to appear in court.

Figure 6-6 A forensic specimen kit such as this one may be used at your facility.

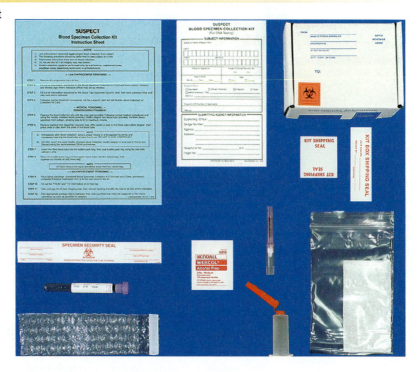

1. If a patient refuses a blood alcohol blood collection, what should you do?

_____

_____

_____

_____

2. What are the general guidelines for collecting a forensic specimen?

_____

_____

_____

_____

Answer the questions above and complete the *Blood Alcohol, Toxicology, and Forensic Specimens* activity on the Student CD under Chapter 6 before you continue to the next section.

6-7 Therapeutic Drug Monitoring

A physician can supervise an individual's drug or medication treatment by using **therapeutic drug monitoring** (TDM). The dosage of medication necessary to produce the desired effect varies with each patient. Drug toxicity must be avoided, and monitoring the level of medicine is one way to establish beneficial levels in each patient. The types of drugs that can be monitored include anticonvulsants, antidepressants, digoxin, lithium, and theophylline (see Table 6-4). Obtaining specimens for drug monitoring requires a routine venipuncture. The difference in therapeutic drug monitoring from other venipunctures is the time of the collection. Timing of specimen collection is critical for drug monitoring. Peak levels are collected when the medicine is at its highest serum concentration, usually 15 to 30 minutes after the drug was administered. Trough levels are collected when the serum concentration is expected to be at its lowest level, usually immediately before administration of the next scheduled dose.

For an inpatient, the phlebotomist should check with the patient's nurse before drawing the specimen to validate that the time is optimal for the levels being tested. It is not uncommon for dosage schedules to get behind due to infiltrated IVs, medications not delivered from the pharmacy in time, or even having the medication discontinued before the scheduled draw time.

Most of the peak and troughs will be ordered on antibiotics that can be toxic at high levels, but ineffective at lower levels. Drugs such as vancomycin, gentamicin, tobramycin, and amikacin have what is known as a short half-life, making the time of collection more critical. Timing is less crucial for those drugs with a longer half-life, such as digoxin and phenobarbital. If the phlebotomist cannot make the draw on time due to a STAT draw in

TABLE 6-4 Common Medications Requiring Therapeutic Monitoring

Medication	Indication
Anticonvulsants (phenobarbital, phenytoin)	• Used to decrease or prevent abnormal discharge of electrical impulse in the central nervous system • Treats seizure activity
Antidepressants (Thorazine)	• Used to elevate the mood of patients • Treats depression
Lanoxin (digoxin)	• Used to increase strength of heart contraction and to slow the rate • Treats heart failure such as congestive heart failure
Lithium	• Stabilizes the patient's mood swings from euphoric and depressed to a stable level • Used to treat manic-depressive psychosis
Theophylline	• Opens respiratory passage (bronchial tubes) so air can pass more freely • Used to treat asthma and bronchitis
Antibiotics (vancomycin, gentamicin, tobramycin, amikacin)	• Used to treat infections
Blood thinners (heparin and warfarin)	• Treatment of heart patients • Treatment of coagulation disorders

another area, the phlebotomist should page someone else to obtain the draw or check with the nurse as soon as possible to see if he or she wants to reschedule the draw around the next dosage times. It is especially important for the phlebotomist to note the times specimens are drawn. In general, peak concentrations are collected when testing for toxicity and trough concentrations alone are useful for demonstrating a good therapeutic concentration. Trough levels are commonly collected for such drugs as lithium, theophylline, phenytoin, carbamazepine, quinidine, valproic acid, and digoxin. It is essential that all specimens are labeled peak and trough.

Checkpoint Questions 6-7

1. When is a peak drug level drawn?

   _____

   _____

   _____

   _____

2. When is a trough drug level drawn?

   _____

   _____

   _____

   _____

Answer the questions above and complete the *Therapeutic Drug Monitoring* activity on the Student CD under Chapter 6 before you continue to the next section.

6-8 Alternative Collection Sites

In addition to venipuncture and capillary puncture, blood may be collected from alternative sites. Venous blood can be collected from a variety of venous access devices that are used on a patient for intravenous therapy and/or blood collection. Arterial blood is collected directly from an artery for special tests that determine the ability of the lungs to exchange oxygen and carbon dioxide.

Venous Access Devices

A venous access device is typically a hollow tube, known as a **cannula,** inserted and left in a vein. The most common type used for obtaining blood samples is commonly known as the heparin lock.

A heparin lock is a special winged needle set that is left in a patient's vein for 48 to 72 hours, depending on institutional policy (see Figure 6-7). A heparin lock is inserted into a patient when obtaining blood is difficult or when a patient must have multiple draws within a short period of time. Licensed practitioners may also use this device to administer certain medications. The cannula, or needle set, must be flushed periodically with

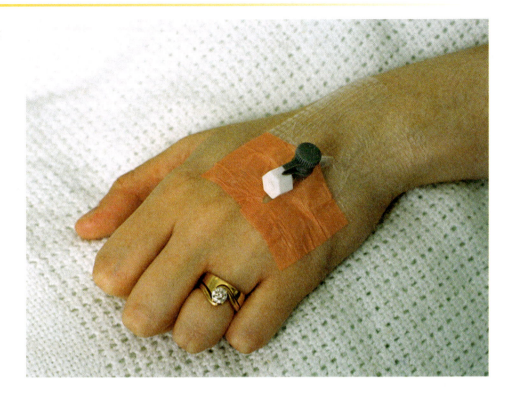

Figure 6-7 A heparin lock may be used to collect blood specimens. This cannula is flushed with normal saline between blood collections to ensure an accurate specimen.

heparin or normal saline, depending on the institution, to keep the lock from clotting. If heparin is used for flushing, the first 5 mL must be discarded before specimens are collected. This is not a procedure normally performed by phlebotomists, and only specially trained personnel should draw blood from a heparin lock assembly, as determined by each facility.

Other types of venous access devices that may be used to collect a specimen include central venous therapy lines and shunts. Central venous therapy is the introduction of a cannula into a vein other than a peripheral vein. Arterial venous shunts are devices inserted into the forearm to allow for hemodialysis. In hemodialysis the shunt is connected to a machine that filters the blood. This is typically done for patients with severe kidney disease. Shunts and central venous lines are not accessed by a phlebotomist to obtain a venous specimen.

Arterial Punctures

An arterial puncture is usually performed to test arterial blood gases (ABGs). ABGs measure the ability of the lungs to exchange oxygen and carbon dioxide. Results of ABGs include the partial pressure of oxygen (PO_2) and carbon dioxide (PCO_2) present in the arterial blood, along with the pH level of the blood. Arterial blood is needed for the assessment of blood gases. A phlebotomist does not normally perform arterial puncture. Special training is required for personnel performing arterial punctures. Arterial puncture training must include the complications associated with arterial puncture, precautions for patient safety, and specimen handling procedures. In many institutions the collecting and performing of arterial punctures has become the responsibility of the respiratory therapy department. Physicians, nurses, medical technologists, respiratory therapists, and other licensed personnel are trained to perform arterial punctures.

Several conditions require the measurement of arterial blood gases. These conditions include chronic obstructive pulmonary disease (COPD), cardiac failure, respiratory failure, severe shock, lung cancer, coronary bypass, open-heart surgery, and respiratory distress syndrome. Usually patients who have arterial blood gases drawn are critically ill. When an arterial specimen is drawn, it must be tested immediately.

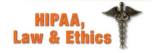

HIPAA, Law & Ethics

Arterial Puncture

It is outside the scope of practice of a phlebotomist to perform an arterial puncture, and it should not be attempted without proper training. If performed improperly a patient could lose the function of a hand. In addition, the risk of infection is greater in arterial punctures, so a cleansing procedure similar to blood culture collection must be employed. Compared to venipuncture, an arterial puncture is far more dangerous to the patient. Many complications can occur, such as hematoma formation, thrombosis, hemorrhage, infection, and permanent nerve damage. Therefore, never attempt an arterial puncture until trained by a professional.

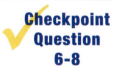

✓ Checkpoint Question 6-8

1. Name four alternative sites that may be used to obtain a blood specimen but are only used by specially trained or licensed individuals.

   _____

   _____

   _____

   _____

   _____

 Answer the question above and complete the *Alternative Collection Sites* activity on the Student CD under Chapter 6 before you continue to the next section.

Chapter Summary

- Specimen collections should be drawn at specified times to ensure accuracy. A patient intake of food, alcohol, tobacco, and medications can affect the results. In addition, posture, exercise, stress, and times of day can affect blood results.
- Two tests that require fasting include various glucose evaluations and triglycerides.
- Various types of glucose tests include fasting blood sugar, 2-hour post-prandial blood sugar, random blood sugar, 2- or 3-hour oral glucose tolerance test, glucose challenge screening test, and intravenous glucose tolerance test.

- The bleeding time test helps assess the ability of platelets to function during a bleeding episode. Situations that can cause a prolonged bleeding time include platelet dysfunction, decreased platelet number, fibrinogen disorders, and medications that hinder platelet functions.
- To obtain blood for donation a phlebotomist must have special training, and the patient must meet certain physician requirements and must submit to a detailed patient interview and mini physical examination.
- Patients may donate blood for their future use. This is known as autologous donation. Other patients may have blood drawn to treat a disease or disorder of the blood. This is known as therapeutic phlebotomy.
- To perform blood alcohol testing the patient must consent or a legal document must be obtained. The site for venipuncture should be cleaned with something other than alcohol.
- A forensic specimen is collected as evidence to help prove or disprove a link between an individual and/or between individuals and objects or places. Toxicology specimens are collected to detect poisons, drugs, or medications.
- Therapeutic drug monitoring is done to ensure the correct amount of drug is given to produce the desired effect.
- Other sites for blood specimen collection include heparin lock, arterial venous shunt, central venous therapy lines, and arterial punctures.

Chapter Review

Multiple Choice

Circle the correct answer.

1. Which of the following can affect glucose levels?
   a. Chewing sugarless gum
   b. Drinking tea or coffee without sugar
   c. Smoking cigarettes
   d. All of the above

2. Which of the following can be used to clean a site before blood alcohol collection?
   a. Isopropanol
   b. Alcohol prep pads
   c. Hydrogen peroxide
   d. Iodine

3. A lipemic specimen is a clue that the patient is:
   a. In a basal state
   b. Smoking cigarettes
   c. Not fasting
   d. Normal

4. What liquid is acceptable to drink when fasting?
   a. Milk
   b. Fruit juice
   c. Black coffee
   d. Water

5. Which of the following tests may require special chain-of-custody documentation?
   a. Therapeutic drug monitoring
   b. Blood culture
   c. Drug screen
   d. Blood donor

6. Which of the following tests is most often a timed specimen?
   a. Toxicology
   b. Triglycerides
   c. Therapeutic drug monitoring
   d. CBC

7. Name a condition in which a unit of blood is drawn from a patient as treatment.
   a. ABO Rh typing
   b. Polycythemia
   c. Leukemia
   d. Anemia

8. The fasting specimen for a GTT is collected:
   a. At 0700
   b. In a lavender-topped tube
   c. While the patient drinks the glucose
   d. And tested before the patient drinks the glucose

9. Which of the following tests is most critical as to exact volume of blood requirements?
   a. Prothrombin
   b. Triglycerides
   c. CBC
   d. Therapeutic drug monitoring

10. A 2-hour PP is often used as a screening test for what condition?
    a. Diabetes
    b. Coagulation problems
    c. Fever of unknown origin
    d. Therapeutic drug monitoring

11. Chilling will affect the test results for which of the following?
    a. Glucose
    b. Ammonia
    c. Prothrombin
    d. Blood culture

12. Which of the following sites is typically used by a phlebotomist to obtain a blood specimen?
    a. Heparin lock
    b. Arterial venous shunt
    c. Antecubital fossa
    d. Central venous line

13. Which of the following tests is commonly done to identify the risk for gestational diabetes?
    a. Random blood sugar
    b. Fasting blood sugar
    c. IVGTT
    d. Glucose challenge test

14. How long must a patient fast for an FBS?
    a. 4 to 6 hours
    b. 2 to 4 hours
    c. 6 to 7 hours
    d. 8 to 12 hours

15. Which of the following is the best reason that a PFA should be done instead of a bleeding time test?
    a. It does not take as long.
    b. It is less painful and more sensitive.
    c. It is easier to perform and less painful.
    d. It is less effective but more sensitive.

Matching

Match each of the key terms to the appropriate definition by placing the correct letter in the spaces provided.

_____ **16.** basal state

_____ **17.** diurnal variation

_____ **18.** fasting

_____ **19.** glycolysis

_____ **20.** hemochromatosis

_____ **21.** peak

_____ **22.** postprandial

_____ **23.** trough

_____ **24.** chain of custody

_____ **25.** analyte

_____ **26.** assay

_____ **27.** lipemic

_____ **28.** bleeding time

_____ **29.** gestational diabetes

_____ **30.** cannula

a. Highest concentration of a drug level

b. Laboratory analysis of a substance

c. After a meal

d. Increased fats in the blood

e. Lowest concentration of a drug level

f. Evaluates platelet function

g. Normal body reaction where glucose is broken down by an enzyme

h. Increased blood sugar during pregnancy

i. Having nothing to eat or drink except water for 8–12 hours

j. 12-hour period without intake of food and exercise

k. Normal daily changes in lab values

l. Disorder of iron metabolism

m. Substance undergoing analysis

n. Hollow tube used for blood access

o. Protocol for document specimen accountability

True or False

Place the letter T in the space provided if you agree that the statement is true or F if the statement is false. For each of the incorrect statements, correct them to make them true.

_____ **31.** A physician's written order is required for anyone who wishes to donate blood.

_____ **32.** One blood donor unit consists of between 450 and 500 milliliters of blood.

_____ **33.** Donors must weigh at least 110 pounds.

_____ **34.** A donor unit containing whole blood can be separated to yield red blood cells, plasma, and platelets.

_____ **35.** Autologous blood is blood donated by a relative.

_____ **36.** Timed specimens are not necessary when it comes to collecting a blood sample.

_____ **37.** Glucose levels aid in diagnosing hepatitis B.

_____ **38.** Hemochromatosis is a disease in which the body stores abnormal amounts of iron.

_____ **39.** Polycythemia is a disease that causes underproduction in the number of red blood cells.

_____ **40.** Arterial punctures are usually drawn from an artery in the wrist.

What Should You Do?

Use your critical-thinking skills to answer the following situations.

41. You are about to draw an out-patient's 2-hour postprandial glucose. She informs you that it has been only one and one-half hours since she ate her lunch. You are on a tight schedule because of the three phlebotomists scheduled to work today, you are the only one who showed up. What would you do?

    _____

    _____

42. As a phlebotomist you're asked to perform arterial blood gases on your first official day as a phlebotomist. You have not had any further training and development. What would be your initial reaction?

    _____

    _____

    _____

    _____

    _____

Get Connected *Internet Activity*

Visit the McGraw-Hill Higher Education Online Learning Center *Phlebotomy for Health Care Personnel* Website at **www.mhhe.com/healthcareskills** to complete the following activity.

1. Visit the American Red Cross Website and research the requirements for donating blood. Create a list of requirements for a donor and reasons why blood should not be collected for transfusion to someone else.

Using the Student CD

Now that you have completed the material in the chapter text, return to the Student CD and complete any chapter activities you have not yet done. Practice your terminology with the "Key Term Concentration" game. Review the chapter material with the "Spin the Wheel" game. Take the final chapter test and complete the troubleshooting question. E-mail or print your results to document your proficiency for this chapter.

7 Practicing Phlebotomy

Learning Outcomes

Upon completion of this chapter, you should be able to:

- Describe certification for phlebotomists.
- Identify the need for phlebotomy continuing education.
- Define quality assurance (QA) as it pertains to phlebotomy.
- Define quality control (QC) as it pertains to phlebotomy.
- List at least three factors that affect laboratory values.
- Identify reasons for specimen rejection.
- Define risk management.
- Describe risk management issues of liability and safety as they relate to phlebotomy.

Key Terms

accreditation

accuracy

American Certification Agency (ACA)

American Medical Technologist (AMT)

American Society of Clinical Pathologists (ASCP)

American Society of Phlebotomy Technicians (ASPT)

calibration

certification

control substance

liability

litigation

malpractice

Material Safety Data Sheets (MSDS)

National Accrediting Agency for Clinical Laboratory Sciences (NAACLS)

National Center for Competency Testing (NCCT)

National Credentialing Agency for Medical Laboratory Personnel (NCA)

National Healthcareer Association (NHA)

outcome

performance improvement

process

quality assurance (QA)

quality control (QC)
quantity not sufficient (QNS)
reliable

risk management
total quality management (TQM)

7-1 Introduction

Once you have completed your education as a phlebotomist you will need to practice in a professional manner. This includes completion of certification and continuing education. As a practicing phlebotomist you are required to provide quality assurance and quality control within your daily duties. Following policies of the institution where you are employed and providing quality specimens are necessary. Most importantly you should have an understanding of risk management including liabilities and safety issues relative to phlebotomy practice.

Checkpoint Question 7-1

1. What are five important areas of knowledge you should have as a phlebotomist?

_____

_____

_____

_____

_____

7-2 Certification and Continuing Education

As mentioned in Chapter 1, the Clinical and Laboratory Standards Institute (CLSI) consists of representatives from the government, industry, and the medical profession. This national nonprofit organization sets standards for phlebotomy training and other laboratory program approval. Questions for certification examinations are based on CLSI standards. Health care professionals are finding it advantageous to have national certification or licensure in their chosen profession, and phlebotomy is no exception. Certified phlebotomists have proven that they understand the standards for their profession. **Certification** is a process that ensures successful completion of defined academic and training requirements and a passing score on a national examination. The purpose of certification is to protect the public by setting standards for individuals working at various levels of responsibility. Licensure, on the other hand, is a process similar to certification, but it applies at the state or local level. A license to practice a specific trade is attained after a person who meets the requirements for education and experience in that trade successfully passes an examination.

In contrast to certification and licensure for individuals, **accreditation** is on a much larger scale. Phlebotomy training programs are evaluated by the **National Accrediting Agency for Clinical Laboratory Sciences (NAACLS)** and other accrediting agencies to ensure that the competencies taught are adequate to provide accurate laboratory results. Accreditation usually has to do with a program of study, not an individual. Accreditation of health care training programs provides individuals assurance of the quality of that program. The accreditation process involves external peer review of the educational program. This includes a written document and onsite inspection to determine if the program meets established qualifications or educational standards referred to as "essentials." The CLSI develops the guidelines and sets standards for all areas of the laboratory, whereas the NAACLS defines essentials for educational programs in the health care field and offers certification for structured educational programs.

After completion of a structured educational program, phlebotomists can take certification exams that meet the standards of the certifying organization. Successful completion of certification requirements validates the individual's ability to perform the program's competencies, or essentials. Successful completion of, or passing, a national examination affords individuals the right to wear a title after their name that signifies credentials. Agencies responsible for providing phlebotomy certification are the **American Certification Agency (ACA)**, the **American Society of Clinical Pathologists (ASCP)**, the **National Credentialing Agency for Medical Laboratory Personnel (NCA)**, the **American Society of Phlebotomy Technicians (ASPT)**, the **National Healthcareer Association (NHA)**, the **National Center for Competency Testing (NCCT)**, and **American Medical Technologists (AMT)**. Certification requirements are becoming the norm for entry-level employment, and although it is not always mandatory, certification is desirable for career advancement. Health care consumers (patients) today look for evidence of competency among all health care workers.

In addition to certification, participation in continuing education assists in establishing a professional public image. Most certifying agencies have specific guidelines regarding how much and what kind of continuing education is required to maintain certification. However, more importantly, as a professional phlebotomist, continuing education is a lifelong process necessary to stay current in your field.

You can continue your education in a variety of ways. Use the Internet to subscribe to learning modules or online tutorials. Many of these can be completed, scored, and sent to your certifying agency directly from your computer. Workshops and seminars are also available and provide interaction with individuals in your field. Staff development programs are available at many health care facilities that provide additional continuing education opportunities. Remember to stay current through education and maintaining membership in professional organizations.

Checkpoint Questions 7-2

1. What is the difference between certification and accreditation?

_____

_____

_____

_____

2. Name three ways you can obtain continuing education.

_____

_____

_____

_____

_____

Answer the questions above and complete the *Certification and Continuing Education* activity on the Student CD under Chapter 7 before you continue to the next section.

7-3 Quality Assurance in Phlebotomy

Total quality management (TQM) is an institutional concept. It involves all members of the health care team creating quality **processes** (actual procedures or duties that are done to the patient) to improve customer satisfaction. This satisfaction is achieved as a result of both the health care encounter and the **accuracy** of the results. For example, as mentioned in Chapter 1, a phlebotomist with an unprofessional appearance and demeanor will adversely affect the patient's satisfaction with services received. Likewise, inaccurate results, for any reason, not only may yield poor patient satisfaction, but may result in medical liability as well. Health care teams are empowered to do more than just the bare minimum. Instead, team members are to monitor and document processes and ensure patient satisfaction. Some health care facilities request patients to complete surveys or other rating systems to ascertain their level of satisfaction with the care they received.

Patients requiring phlebotomy services evaluate the care they receive not just on their lab results but also on the following factors:

- How long they had to wait for the procedure
- The presence or absence of bruising to the site
- How many needlesticks or attempts were required
- Their perception of the phlebotomist (e.g., dress, communication skill)

Patients who have to wait a minimum amount of time for their blood to be drawn with only one needlestick and who encounter a well-groomed, professional phlebotomist will generally rate their experience with positive marks.

Quality assurance (QA) is a system for evaluating performance, as in the delivery of services or the quality of products provided to consumers, customers, or patients. This system is set forth to guarantee quality patient care by continued reassessment of all processes.

Quality assurance refers to planned, step-by-step activities that let one know that testing is being carried out correctly, results are accurate, and mistakes are found and corrected to avoid adverse outcomes. Quality assurance is an ongoing set of activities that help to ensure that the test results provided are as accurate and reliable as possible for all persons being tested. Quality assurance activities should be in place during the entire testing process; this means from the time a person asks to be tested until the results are documented and logged into the system.

Laboratory tests are a vital link that assists physicians in identifying a patient's medical diagnosis. Quality performance, starting with the physician's order and the phlebotomist and continuing until the specimen results are obtained, is imperative to quality patient care. A certain level of quality must exist at all stages, from the completed lab requisition to specimen processing, in order for the results to be accurate. This level of quality must be consistently present throughout the entire process. Physicians and patients rely on laboratory team members for such quality performance.

The assessment of any process requires the establishment of indicators, such as those presented in Figure 7-1, that are measurable, specific, well-defined, and essential to the process. Indicators are designed to assess areas of care that tend to cause problems or negative **outcomes** (results). They measure quality, accuracy, timeliness, customer satisfaction, and adequacy, to name a few. An example of an indicator on a facility laboratory quality assessment form would be as follows: "Wristband identification errors will be less than 1%." In order to evaluate such an indicator, specific, scheduled evaluations of various documents such as patient records, incident reports, lab reports, and direct patient observations may be used. By reviewing available data, indicators can be evaluated.

Evaluation is to show not only outcomes but processes as well. Using the sample indicator just mentioned, if the number of wristband identification errors were to exceed 1%, a numerical value would represent this. Knowing that the number of wristband identification errors exceeds the

Figure 7-1 In the phlebotomy chain of accountability for laboratory tests, the phlebotomist will be responsible for numbers 3, 4, 5, and 6 of the nine chain links listed, and perhaps all nine, depending on the place of employment.

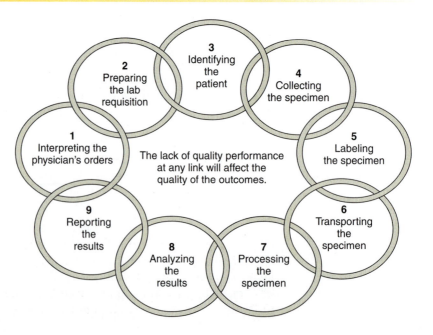

acceptable level will not provide a solution to the problem. If, however, the entire process is reviewed, the results of each step in the process could be evaluated for flaws. Most patients would assume that the cause of such a problem would be the failure of the phlebotomist to check the wristband. However, in this example the hospital admitting clerk, the health care personnel caring for the patient, and the phlebotomist drawing the blood would all be vital checkpoints that might yield another cause for such an unwanted outcome. The process of evaluating each procedural step for accuracy is another component of quality assurance commonly referred to as **quality control (QC)**.

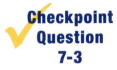

Checkpoint Question 7-3

1. In addition to laboratory results, what other factors would be evaluated for quality assurance?

_____

_____

_____

_____

Answer the question above and complete the *Quality Assurance in Phlebotomy* activity on the Student CD under Chapter 7 before you continue to the next section.

Patient Education & Communication

Informing Patients

Certain blood tests, such as plasma cortisol levels, are affected by diurnal variations (meaning they will yield different results based on the time of day they are drawn) and by whether the patient has been moving around. Hospitalized and outpatients must have such lab tests drawn at the same time to ensure quality results. Plasma cortisol levels drawn around 3:00 P.M. will be much lower—about half the value—than levels drawn between 7:00 A.M. and 9:00 A.M. This information should be shared with patients so they will understand the importance of adhering to scheduled times for their blood levels to be drawn. Quality assurance programs ensure that policies and procedures are available to address instances such as this so that quality results are guaranteed.

7-4 Quality Control in Phlebotomy

Quality control examines individual steps in the whole process to guarantee quality patient outcomes. Accuracy is essential if quality results are expected. Normal parameters are established for all laboratory tests, especially point-of-care testing (POCT), as discussed in Chapter 5, in order to evaluate the outcomes. Basically, quality control measures ensure that procedural steps are followed and yield consistent results. Thus, quality control monitors the testing process and quality assurance measures patient outcomes. Once variances are identified, corrective action plans can be implemented and monitored for improvement. Evaluating the whole process is essential, especially with laboratory tests. Laboratory tests require preparation of both the equipment and the patient prior to specimen collection. In order to obtain an appropriate specimen, the patient must have been properly prepared. Various tests require different types of preparation. Health care facilities have instruction manuals that describe special preparations and collection procedures that must be followed. This manual is referred to as the laboratory user or procedure manual, and the contents are to ensure compliance with JCAHO, CLIA, and other regulatory agency guidelines. This manual must be available for all health care personnel involved in the specimen collection process to use as a reference. Failure to adhere to the laboratory user manual can adversely affect the quality of the specimen obtained and may therefore alter the results.

Troubleshooting

Using Quality Assurance Resources

If a patient is scheduled to have a plasma cortisol level drawn at 9:00 A.M. but the patient does not arrive for the blood work until 3:00 P.M., the phlebotomist should notify the licensed practitioner immediately. It is very likely that the physician will request that the test be rescheduled for the following day because of the diurnal variations associated with plasma cortisol levels. The laboratory quality assurance policy and procedure manual should provide instructions for handling such situations. Other substances affected by diurnal variations are hormone levels, serum iron, and serum glucose levels.

Question: What document helps the phlebotomist make decisions on the job?

_____

_____

_____

Quality Control Activities

Quality control activities may include a check of supplies to ensure that they are not outdated or damaged; the **calibration,** or adjustment, of equipment; and the performance of function checks, to name a few (see Figure 7-2). Prior to using POCT equipment such as a glucometer, a control check is performed to validate the accuracy of the testing system. For example, calibration results may yield 80 mg/dL when the system is checked, yet the correct written reading should be 90 mg/dL. This means the system must be adjusted to the acceptable reading of 90 mg/dL before using the equipment for patient testing. Some adjustments are made manually, whereas newer systems detect changes electronically and automatically make the necessary adjustments without operator assistance. The **control substance,** whether liquid, serum,

Figure 7-2 Quality control records are maintained on equipment to ensure accuracy of test results.

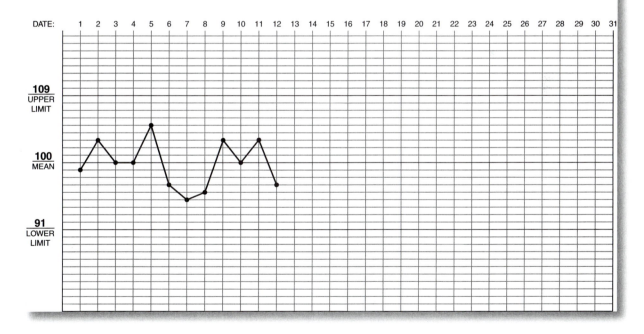

QUALITY CONTROL RECORD

PRACTICE NAME
PRECISION HEALTH CARE INC.

DEPARTMENT	**Glucose Monitor-Institution #55**					NAME/LEVEL
CONTROL LOT #	**H542A**		EXPIRATION DATE	**01/29/XX**		
DIRECTOR SIGNATURE DATE:						

TEST											UNITS
LOWER LIMIT				MEAN				UPPER LIMIT			
DATE	No.	VALUE	TECH	COMMENT	DATE	No.	VALUE	TECH	COMMENT		
12/8/XX	1	99	KBH			17					
12/9/XX	2	103	KBH	prev. maintenance		18					
12/10/XX	3	100	KBH			19					
12/11/XX	4	100	KBH			20					
12/14/XX	5	105	KBH			21					
12/15/XX	6	97	KBH			22					
12/16/XX	7	95	KBH			23					
12/17/XX	8	96	KBH	new battery		24					
12/18/XX	9	103	KBH			25					
12/19/XX	10	100	KBH			26					
12/20/XX	11	103	KBH			27					
12/21/XX	12	97	KBH			28					
	13					29					
	14					30					
	15					31					
	16										

or freeze-dried material, has a known value and has been prepared and tested by the manufacturer. This substance or device is used when doing a system check on the equipment. If the readings from the control check are not within the set acceptable parameters, the equipment will not yield accurate results. For example, a test system may have both a high control and a low control with an acceptable range for each, or a test system may have high, low, and normal controls, each with an acceptable range. Values obtained during a system check that fall outside the established parameters warrant immediate repair, calibration, or replacement of the system.

Another important quality control activity is validating that the results obtained will yield the same or similar results if the test is repeated. In other words, if you were to obtain a glucose result of 107 mg/dL, the same or similar value must be obtained if the test were repeated several times by different health care personnel on that same patient. Both accuracy and reproducibility are required quality control checks of equipment if the results are to be **reliable** (believable and dependable). If your results do not match previous results, expected results, or the patient's clinical symptoms, then the test should be repeated.

Yet another quality control activity is documentation of testing. All quality control tests are logged or documented. All patient results are included in the clinical record. These log records are usually maintained for at least two years.

Factors Affecting Laboratory Values

Many factors can affect laboratory values. Test results can be affected by these factors. Some are under the control of the phlebotomist, whereas others are not. However, the phlebotomist should be aware of the following factors:

- Potassium, phosphorus, enzyme levels, and lactate blood levels can be affected by prolonged tourniquet placement.
- The dietary state of the patient is under the phlebotomist's control. Of course, a phlebotomist cannot really control whether or not a person eats, but the phlebotomist *can* control whether or not a person has blood collected. If a specimen has been ordered as fasting, it is up to the phlebotomist to ask the patient if he or she has had anything to eat or drink, except water, for the specified period of time and to make a notation on the lab slip. The patient may say, "No, I haven't had anything to eat or drink," not realizing that even a single cup of coffee can dramatically change test results. A phlebotomist must be specific when asking this question so the patient will not accidentally cause a wrong result.
- Results can be changed if an incorrect volume of blood is drawn into the tube. Too much blood in some tubes will cause clotting. Citrate tubes for coagulation tests are the most critical as to exact volume requirements. Any variation greater than 10 percent can cause variation in coagulation results. In hematology, lavender or EDTA tubes must be filled to at least three-fourths of the total amount; any less will cause the cells to decrease in size and will yield erroneous results. If a gray-topped tube is less than three-fourths full, the potassium oxalate can make the red blood cells swell and rupture, causing hemolysis in the sample. When not enough blood has been collected the specimen is **QNS** (quantity not sufficient).
- The order of draw is the most overlooked cause of erroneous test results. If an EDTA tube is drawn before a citrate tube, for example, the PT and APTT results will be erroneously increased.
- Some tests require that the sample be chilled immediately after collection, such as ammonia and HLA-B27. Any delay in chilling will alter test results.

Specimen Rejection

The collection of a specimen does not necessarily mean that it will undergo processing. If the specimen obtained does not meet specified criteria, the specimen will be rejected. The following are reasons for rejecting collected specimens:

- Specimens lacking proper identification
- Hemolyzed blood sample
- Incorrect tube for specimen
- Improper handling of specimen
- Contamination of specimen
- Inadequate sample to perform test, referred to as "quantity not sufficient" (QNS)
- Incorrect time of specimen collection
- Outdated equipment
- Clotted specimens in an anticoagulated tube
- No date or time marked on the label
- Label information does not match the requisition

Any or all of the above examples are grounds for rejecting the specimen and requiring repeat specimen collection procedures. Events requiring that lab tests be repeated are monitored and assessed using quality control guidelines. The negative outcomes of each event (rejection of the specimen requiring repeat specimen collection) will be evaluated by quality assurance protocols. In some cases only the phlebotomist will know of some of the above conditions. It is an ethical responsibility to let the lab know if possible redraw of a specimen is needed.

Checkpoint Questions 7-4

1. Name three quality control activities.

_____

_____

_____

_____

_____

2. Name at least three conditions or factors that can affect the laboratory value.

_____

_____

_____

_____

Answer the questions above and complete the *Quality Control in Phlebotomy* activity on the Student CD under Chapter 7 before you continue to the next section.

7-5 Risk Management

An enormous amount of potential for injury exists in health care facilities. Such events or occurrences fall under the area of risk management. **Risk management** departments generate policies and procedures to protect patients, employees, and the employer from loss or injury. In addition to issues of safety, hospital risk management departments may also provide policies and procedures designed to protect the institution from **liability,** or legal obligation to compensate for loss or damages, and **litigation,** or legal action.

Patient Issues

Patients are susceptible to numerous risks when they enter a health care facility, from minor falls to the unjustifiable loss of a limb. However, our focus will deal strictly with losses related to phlebotomy. Venipuncture procedures, if improperly performed, can cause temporary or permanent injury to the extremity.

The CLSI has specific standards that apply to all persons who perform venipuncture. This standard provides guidelines for accurate and safe performance of phlebotomy procedures. Most injuries resulting from phlebotomy procedures fall under **malpractice** (incorrect treatment of a patient by a health care worker) or negligence (failure to perform reasonably expected duties to patients) (see Table 7-1). As discussed in Chapter 1, failure to secure the patient's consent for a procedure could result in charges of assault or battery.

Litigation related to health care issues has increased. Today, patients are considered health care consumers. Therefore, they possess a certain level of knowledge and expect a certain level of service to be provided. In the event a patient thinks negligence or malpractice has occurred, the patient is required to prove that such events took place. The health care facility is not required to prove that malpractice or negligence did not occur. The burden of proof is always the responsibility of the patient.

Preventing Liability Suits

All health care personnel must understand and exercise their legal duty to the patient. Phlebotomists must be aware of the standards of care, as well as boundaries and limitations of practice, for phlebotomists. Attempting to perform procedures that you are not fully trained to perform can lead to poor-quality care and perceived negligence. Other health team members

TABLE 7-1 Common Causes of Liability for Phlebotomists

- Misidentification of the patient
- Breach of confidentiality
- Improperly labeled specimens
- Performing venipuncture without consent
- Injury to blood vessels or nerves
- Poor sterile technique resulting in patient infection
- Permanent scarring or disfigurement
- Acting outside scope of practice (for example, helping a patient to the restroom and the patient falls and is injured)
- Starting an IV or performing ABGs
- Mishandling a specimen, resulting in misdiagnosis or erroneous treatment

may attempt to delegate tasks, such as arterial puncture, that go beyond the phlebotomist's level of training and expertise. Never perform any procedures you are not fully trained to perform. Many health care facilities cross-train employees to perform skills they were not formally trained to do in their educational programs. All persons performing phlebotomy, whether formally trained or cross-trained, must do so according to the established standard of care to prevent potential litigation.

HIPAA, Law & Ethics

4 Ds of Medical Malpractice

For a lawsuit involving medical malpractice, the plaintiff, or patient bringing the lawsuit, must prove that the defendant or phlebotomist facing the charges:

- Owed a *duty* or the patient was being treated by the phlebotomist.
- Was *derelict,* or in other words did not live up to the obligation of caring for the patient.
- Committed a breach of duty of care that was direct cause of *damages* to the patient.
- Is *due* to (or a direct result of) the treatment by the phlebotomist.

Since blood collection is an invasive procedure, you are at risk for injuring a patient. However, with proper training and supervision your risk is reduced. Always follow the standards of care at your facility (use the laboratory procedure manual) and do not work outside your scope of practice. You will want to obtain malpractice insurance in case an incident occurs.

Avoidance of destructive and unethical criticism of other team members is a must. Patients hearing negative comments about other team members may develop negative perceptions about that team member and the facility before they ever interact with them. Never discuss a former practitioner or other team member involving a negative experience with patients. Allow patients to discuss their concerns, but do not add comments to the discussion that might be construed as an admission of fault.

As discussed in Chapter 1, communication must be done with tact and professionalism when handling patients. In the event a patient discloses to you any dissatisfaction with a practitioner or other team member, discuss this with the appropriate person so the problem can be rectified. Do not lead the patient to believe that this disclosed information will be kept confidential, because addressing customer concerns is important in limiting litigations.

Proper documentation is another vital link to preventing liability. Remember to properly record results or variances immediately to prevent errors and liability. Documentation serves as a blueprint of the health care facility's account of the patient's care and treatment. Good record keeping is often the only account of an event that health care facilities can rely on when faced with potential liability. The patient record is also a communication medium used by the health team members when planning and evaluating care. Each member is responsible for properly documenting essential information.

Several measures are taken by health care personnel to prevent patient injuries and thus reduce liability. The same determination must be exercised to prevent employee injuries and exposure to bloodborne pathogens.

Health Care Personnel Issues

Exposure to bloodborne pathogens presents a great risk to health care employees. Phlebotomists must adhere to CDC and OSHA guidelines. As discussed in Chapter 1, OSHA identified the practice of standard precautions and use of PPEs (masks, gown, and such) to be worn when potential exposure to bloodborne and other pathogens is likely. In addition, OSHA mandated that all health care institutions maintain exposure plans, which are prepared by each institution. These exposure action plans are to serve not only as a step-by-step guide for the employee to follow in the event of exposure, but also as documentation of the event and as recommendation for course of treatment. All employees at risk of exposure to bloodborne pathogens are to be given, free of charge, the hepatitis B vaccination, according to OSHA guidelines.

The actual regulations and mandates from OSHA and the CDC are a small component to preventing exposures. Phlebotomists are at risk with every venipuncture procedure; therefore, safety measures must be taken at all times. The phlebotomist must properly apply PPEs and dispose of all sharps (needles and such) correctly in the designated biohazard containers.

Troubleshooting Exposure Incident

A phlebotomist can follow all institutional policies and procedures and still find himself or herself exposed to bloodborne pathogens. An exposure incident occurs when you accidentally get blood or other potentially infectious material (OPIM) into a break in the skin or mucous membrane. In addition to immediate handwashing and/or flushing of the area, documentation of the occurrence should be filed, along with following other steps on the facility's post-exposure policy. Many health care facilities have occupational health departments that would handle such events.

Question: Name two situations that could cause an exposure incident for a phlebotomist.

_____

_____

_____

Another issue of safety in the laboratory is the presence of various chemicals and substances that could be potentially hazardous. Identification of chemicals that are potentially hazardous is governed by a branch of OSHA called the OSHA Hazardous Communication Standard (OSHA HazCom). This standard requires labeling of all essential information about the chemical and the presence of **material safety data sheets (MSDS),** which provide precautionary and emergency information about the chemical product (see Figure 7-3). The MSDS manual provides emergency information for immediate treatment, in the event of a spill or splash of a chemical. These sheets also indicate specific data about each substance, such as if it is flammable, what other agents react with it, and how to dispose of the substance, to name a few. Phlebotomists must be familiar with all potential hazards to ensure their safety.

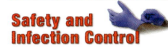

Safety and Infection Control

Cleaning Up Spills

The laboratory has plenty of substances that have the potential to be spilled. When a spill occurs make sure you are trained and know the correct procedure for cleaning up the material. In some cases you may need to check the material safety data sheets or the laboratory procedure manual. In all cases, use great care and safety when responding to a substance spill. Use a chemical spills kit, if appropriate. These should be kept in a handy location. Handle blood and other potentially infectious materials (OPIM) using standard precautions.

Spills can be prevented or minimized by:

1. Maintaining a neat and organized work area
2. Performing a laboratory procedure review prior to conducting new procedures
3. Keeping reagent chemical containers sealed or closed at all times, except when removing contents
4. Ordering reagent chemicals in plastic or plastic-coated glass containers whenever possible

Checkpoint Questions 7-5

1. What is the difference between malpractice and negligence?

_____

_____

_____

_____

2. Name at least three common causes of liability for the phlebotomist.

_____

_____

_____

_____

3. When might you use an MSDS?

_____

_____

_____

_____

 Answer the questions above and complete the *Risk Management* activity on the Student CD under Chapter 7 before you continue to the next section.

MATERIAL SAFETY DATA SHEET 5,929

05/07/xx

SECTION I — NAME AND PRODUCT

MFG NAME AND ADDRESS		
BBL DIV OF BIOQUEST	CHEMICAL NUMBER	: L31591
P O BOX 243	ITEM NUMBER	: 421525
	VNDR CATLG NBR	:
	ENTRY DATE	: 09-17-xx
COCKEYSVILLE	CHANGE DATE	: 01-09-xx
MD 21030	EMERGENCY PHONE	: 301 8660100

CHEMICAL NAME
SENSI-DISCS CEFOXITIN 20MCO PK/10 CART

TRADE NAME SYN :
SAME AS ABOVE
CHEMICAL FAMILY :
ANTIBIOTIC SUSCEPTIBILITY DISC

SECTION II — HAZARDOUS INGREDIENTS

HAZARDOUS COMPONENTS:
NONE LISTED UNDER OSHA...
THIS PRODUCT CONTAINS ANTIBIOTIC WHICH MAY BE SENSITIZING AND THEREFORE SHOULD NOT COME IN CONTACT WITH SKIN OR EYES. IN ADDITION IT SHOULD NOT BE INGESTED:.....................................NEGLIGIBLE

SECTION III — PHYSICAL DATE S/10 – SEE SECTION X

BOIL POINT	SPECIFIC GRAVITY	VAPOR PRESS.	MELT. POINT	VAPOR DENSITY	EVAP. RATE	SOLUBLE IN WATER	PERCENT VOLATILE
N/A	N/A	N/A	N/A	N/A	N/A	N/A	NEG.
					N/A		

APPEARANCE AND ODOR:
NO DISTINCT ODOR: PAPER DISC

SECTION IV — FIRE AND EXPLOSION HAZARD DATA

FLASH POINT: N/A
FLAMMABLE LEL: N/A
FLAMMABLE UEL: N/A

EXTINGUISHING MEDIA:
DRY CHEMICAL, OR WATER

SPECIAL FIRE FIGHTING PROCEDURES:
N/A

UNUSUAL FIRE AND EXPLOSION HAZARDS:
N/A

Chapter Summary

- Certification ensures successful completion of an examination by a certifying body and protects the public by setting standards for phlebotomy practice.
- Phlebotomy continuing education is necessary to ensure knowledge and skills are up to date and also to meet certification requirements.
- Quality assurance (QA) is a system set forth to guarantee quality patient care by evaluating processes. In phlebotomy, quality performance is necessary from the time the order is written until the results are reported to the patient.
- Quality control (QC) ensures accuracy by establishing standards for procedures, requiring calibration of equipment, validating results, and maintaining accurate documentation.

- Factors that affect laboratory values include extended tourniquet use, incorrect dietary state for tests performed, incorrect volume of blood, incorrect order of the draw, and improper handling of a specimen once collected.
- Specimen rejection can occur for a variety of reasons, including improper identification, hemolysis or coagulation, incorrect tube or handling, contamination, QNS, incorrect time or outdated equipment, date and time of collection not marked, or label information does not match the specimen.
- Risk management identifies policies and procedures to protect patients, employees, and the employer from loss or injury.
- Phlebotomists should work within their scope of practice, following established policies to prevent malpractice. Phlebotomists must follow standard precautions and utilize MSDS information when necessary.

Chapter Review

Matching

Match each term with the correct definition by writing the appropriate letter in the space provided.

_____ **1.** QA

_____ **2.** TCM

_____ **3.** risk management

_____ **4.** QC

_____ **5.** MSDS

_____ **6.** QNS

_____ **7.** accreditation

_____ **8.** certification

a. Quantity not sufficient

b. Creates policies and procedures to protect patients, employees, and employers from loss or injury

c. Examines each procedural step for accuracy

d. Institutional concept involving all members to create quality processes and improve customer satisfaction

e. Educational program requirement

f. Individual educational requirements

g. Program of established policies and procedures that govern all activities of the health care facility

h. Information about each chemical and emergency instructions in the event of exposure

True or False

Write T or F in the blank to indicate whether you think the statement is true or false. Correct each of the false statements to make them true.

_____ **9.** Customer satisfaction regarding health care services relates only to clinical services provided.

_____ **10.** Processes are activities health care providers do for the patient.

_____ **11.** JCAHO mandated that ongoing evaluations be performed by each department in health care facilities.

_____ **12.** Processes are actual procedures that are done to a patient to improve customer satisfaction.

_____ **13.** Clinical indicators are determined by the CDC.

_____ **14.** A gray-topped tube that is not full might cause potassium elevation and will be rejected.

_____ **15.** If a patient ate before a fasting blood test, blood should not be collected.

Fill in the Blanks

Fill in the blanks with the correct word to complete the sentence accurately.

16. The _____ has specified standards that apply to any person performing venipuncture.

17. _____ is the incorrect treatment of a patient by a health care worker.

18. The identification of chemicals that are potentially hazardous is governed by _____.

19. Phlebotomists must follow institutional guidelines, which are in line with both _____ and _____ to prevent exposure to bloodborne pathogens.

20. Acting outside your _____ is a common cause of liability.

21. _____ is an institution-wide concept that involves all members of the health care team in creating quality processes to improve customer satisfaction.
    a. Quality assurance
    b. Quality management
    c. Quality improvements
    d. None of the above

22. Achieving complete correctness or acceptable measures as close as possible to the true value is known as _____.
    a. Calibration
    b. Accuracy
    c. Process
    d. None of the above

23. _____ is the actual procedure or duty that is to be done to the patient.
    a. Reliable
    b. Process
    c. Outcome
    d. None of the above

24. _____ is a nongovernmental, voluntary organization responsible for establishing operational standards for hospitals and other health facilities and services.
    a. OSHA
    b. DHHS
    c. JCAHO
    d. None of the above

25. The _____, whether liquid, serum, or freeze-dried materials, has a known value and has been prepared and tested by the manufacturer.
    a. Calibration
    b. Control substance
    c. Testing agents
    d. Analytes

What Should You Do?

Use your critical thinking skills to respond to the following scenarios.

26. A patient has arrived at 2:00 P.M. for a plasma cortisol level that was scheduled for 8:30 A.M. Should the phlebotomist proceed and draw this blood sample? How could this situation affect the quality of the patient's results?

_____

_____

27. You are performing a routine quality control check on the glucometer machine prior to using it. The machine function check was fine with the low control check, and the high control check reading was 90. The machine you are using has a high control value of 110 mg/dL with an acceptable range of 105–115 mg/dL and a low control value of 75 mg/dL with an acceptable range of 70–80 mg/dL. Determine what actions, if any, are required.

_____

_____

Get Connected *Internet Activity*

Visit the McGraw-Hill Higher Education Online Learning Center *Phlebotomy for Health Care Personnel* Website at **www.mhhe.com/healthcareskills** to complete the following activities:

1. Search the U.S. Department of Labor Occupational Safety and Health Administration to view a sample copy of an exposure control plan. Review the exposure control plan and be prepared to discuss in class.
2. Visit the Web links of the agencies responsible for phlebotomy certification. Review the requirements for certification and continuing education and determine the agency to pursue certification with based upon your qualifications and educational program.

Using the Student CD

Now that you have completed the material in the chapter text, return to the Student CD and complete any chapter activities you have not yet done. Practice your terminology with the "Key Term Concentration" game. Review the chapter material with the "Spin the Wheel" game. Take the final chapter test and complete the troubleshooting question. E-mail or print your results to document your proficiency for this chapter.

Standard Precautions*

Standard Precautions synthesize the major features of Universal Precautions (designed to reduce the risk of transmission of bloodborne pathogens) and Body Substance Isolation (designed to reduce the risk of transmission of pathogens from moist body substances), and applies them to all patients receiving care in hospitals, regardless of their diagnosis or presumed infection status. Standard Precautions apply to the following:

- Blood
- All body fluids, secretions, and excretions except sweat, regardless of whether or not they contain visible blood
- Nonintact skin
- Mucous membranes

Standard Precautions are designed to reduce the risk of transmission of microorganisms from both recognized and unrecognized sources of infection in hospitals. Use Standard Precautions, or the equivalent, for the care of all patients, including the following areas of practice:

A. Handwashing

B. Gloves

C. Mask, eye protection, face shield

D. Gown

E. Patient care equipment

F. Environmental control

G. Linen

H. Occupational health and bloodborne pathogens

I. Patient placement

A. Handwashing

1. Wash hands after touching blood, body fluids, secretions, excretions, and contaminated items, whether or not gloves are worn. Wash hands immediately after gloves are removed, between patient contacts, and when otherwise indicated to avoid transfer of microorganisms to other patients or environments. It may be necessary to wash hands between tasks and procedures on the same patient to prevent cross-contamination of different body sites.

*Adapted from the Occupational Safety and Health Administration Bloodborne Pathogens – 1910.1030 (www.osha.gov).

2. Use a plain (nonantimicrobial) soap for routine handwashing.

3. Use an antimicrobial agent or a waterless antiseptic agent for specific circumstances (e.g., control of outbreaks or hyperendemic infections), as defined by the infection control program. (See Contact Precautions for additional recommendations on using antimicrobial and antiseptic agents.)

B. Gloves

Wear gloves (clean, nonsterile gloves are adequate) when touching blood, body fluids, secretions, excretions, and contaminated items. Put on clean gloves just before touching mucous membranes and nonintact skin. Change gloves between tasks and procedures on the same patient after contact with material that may contain a high concentration of microorganisms. Remove gloves promptly after use, before touching noncontaminated items and environmental surfaces, and before going to another patient, and wash hands immediately to avoid transfer of microorganisms to other patients or environments.

C. Mask, Eye Protection, Face Shield

Wear a mask and eye protection or a face shield to protect mucous membranes of the eyes, nose, and mouth during procedures and patient-care activities that are likely to generate splashes or sprays of blood, body fluids, secretions, and excretions.

D. Gown

Wear a gown (a clean, nonsterile gown is adequate) to protect skin and to prevent soiling of clothing during procedures and patient-care activities that are likely to generate splashes or sprays of blood, body fluids, secretions, or excretions. Select a gown that is appropriate for the activity and amount of fluid likely to be encountered. Remove a soiled gown as promptly as possible, and wash hands to avoid transfer of microorganisms to other patients or environments.

E. Patient-Care Equipment

Handle used patient-care equipment soiled with blood, body fluids, secretions, and excretions in a manner that prevents skin and mucous membrane exposures, contamination of clothing, and transfer of microorganisms to other patients and environments. Ensure that reusable equipment is not used for the care of another patient until it has been cleaned and reprocessed appropriately. Ensure that single-use items are discarded properly.

F. Environmental Control

Ensure that the hospital has adequate procedures for the routine care, cleaning, and disinfection of environmental surfaces, beds, bedrails, bedside equipment, and other frequently touched surfaces, and ensure that these procedures are being followed.

G. Linen

Handle, transport, and process used linen soiled with blood, body fluids, secretions, and excretions in a manner that prevents skin and mucous membrane exposures and contamination of clothing, and that avoids transfer of microorganisms to other patients and environments.

H. Occupational Health and Bloodborne Pathogens

1. Take care to prevent injuries when using needles, scalpels, and other sharp instruments or devices; when handling sharp instruments after procedures; when cleaning used instruments; and when disposing of used needles. Never recap used needles, or otherwise manipulate them using both hands, or use any other technique that involves directing the point of a needle toward any part of the body; rather, use either a one-handed "scoop" technique or a mechanical device designed for holding the needle sheath. Do not remove used needles from disposable syringes by hand, and do not bend, break, or otherwise manipulate used needles by hand. Place used disposable syringes and needles, scalpel blades, and other sharp items in appropriate puncture-resistant containers, which are located as close as practical to the area in which the items were used, and place reusable syringes and needles in a puncture-resistant container for transport to the reprocessing area.

2. Use mouthpieces, resuscitation bags, or other ventilation devices as an alternative to mouth-to-mouth resuscitation methods in areas where the need for resuscitation is predictable.

I. Patient Placement

Place a patient who contaminates the environment or who does not (or cannot be expected to) assist in maintaining appropriate hygiene or environmental control in a private room. If a private room is not available, consult with infection control professionals regarding patient placement or other alternatives.

B Appendix

Transmission-Based Precautions*

There are three categories of Transmission-Based Precautions:

1. Contact Precautions
2. Droplet Precautions
3. Airborne Precautions

Transmission-Based Precautions are used when the route(s) of transmission is (are) not completely interrupted using Standard Precautions alone. For some diseases that have multiple routes of transmission (e.g., SARS), more than one Transmission-Based Precautions category may be used. When used either singly or in combination, they are always used in addition to Standard Precautions.

Contact Precautions

Contact Precautions are intended to prevent transmission of infectious agents, including important microorganisms, which are spread by direct or indirect contact with the patient or the patient's environment. Certain infections require the use of Contact Precautions, including patients infected or colonized with multidrug-resistant organisms. Contact Precautions also apply where the presence of excessive wound drainage, fecal incontinence, or other discharges from the body suggest an increased potential for extensive environmental contamination and risk of transmission. A single-patient room is preferred for patients who require Contact Precautions. When a single-patient room is not available, consultation with infection control personnel is recommended to assess the various risks associated with other patient placement options (e.g., cohorting, keeping the patient with an existing roommate). In multi-patient rooms, at least 3 feet of spatial separation between beds is advised to reduce the opportunities for inadvertent sharing of items between the infected/colonized patient and other patients. Health care personnel caring for patients on Contact Precautions wear a gown and gloves for all interactions that may involve contact with the patient or potentially contaminated areas in the patient's environment. Donning PPE upon room entry and discarding before exiting the patient room is done to contain pathogens, especially those that have been implicated in transmission through environmental contamination such as vancomycin-resistant enterococci, *C. difficile,* noroviruses, and other intestinal tract pathogens.

*Adapted from Centers for Disease Control Guidelines for Isolation Precautions 2007 (www.cdc.gov).

Droplet Precautions

Droplet Precautions are intended to prevent transmission of pathogens spread through close respiratory or mucous membrane contact with respiratory secretions. Because these pathogens do not remain infectious over long distances in a health care facility, special air handling and ventilation are not required to prevent droplet transmission. Infectious agents for which Droplet Precautions are indicated include *pertussis,* influenza virus, adenovirus, rhinovirus, *N. meningitides,* and group A streptococcus (for the first 24 hours of antimicrobial therapy). A single-patient room is preferred for patients who require Droplet Precautions. When a single-patient room is not available, consultation with infection control personnel is recommended to assess the various risks associated with other patient placement options (e.g., cohorting, keeping the patient with an existing roommate). Spatial separation of at least 3 feet and drawing the curtain between patient beds is especially important for patients in multi-bed rooms with infections transmitted by the droplet route. Health care personnel wear a mask (a respirator is not necessary) for close contact with infectious patients; the mask is generally donned upon room entry. Patients on Droplet Precautions who must be transported outside of the room should wear a mask if tolerated and follow Respiratory Hygiene/Cough Etiquette.

Airborne Precautions

Airborne Precautions prevent transmission of infectious agents that remain infectious over long distances when suspended in the air (e.g., rubeola virus [measles], varicella virus [chickenpox], *M. tuberculosis*, and possibly SARS-CoV). The preferred placement for patients who require Airborne Precautions is in an airborne infection isolation room (AIIR). An AIIR is a single-patient room that is equipped with special air handling and ventilation capacity that meet the American Institute of Architects/Facility Guidelines Institute (AIA/FGI) standards for AIIRs. Some states require the availability of such rooms in hospitals, emergency departments, and nursing homes that care for patients with *M. tuberculosis*. A respiratory protection program that includes education about use of respirators, fit-testing, and user seal checks is required in any facility with AIIRs. In settings where Airborne Precautions cannot be implemented due to limited engineering resources (e.g., physician offices), masking the patient, placing the patient in a private room (e.g., office examination room) with the door closed, and providing N95 or higher level respirators or masks if respirators are not available for health care personnel will reduce the likelihood of airborne transmission until the patient is either transferred to a facility with an AIIR or returned to the home environment, as deemed medically appropriate. Health care personnel caring for patients on Airborne Precautions wear a mask or respirator mask that is donned prior to room entry. Whenever possible, non-immune health care workers should not care for patients with vaccine-preventable airborne diseases (e.g., measles, chickenpox, and smallpox).

Applications of Transmission-Based Precautions

Diagnosis of many infections requires laboratory confirmation. Since laboratory tests, especially those that depend on culture techniques, often require two or more days for completion, Transmission-Based Precautions must be implemented while test results are pending based on the clinical presentation and likely pathogens. Use of appropriate Transmission-Based Precautions at the time a patient develops symptoms or signs of transmissible infection, or arrives at a health care facility for care, reduces transmission opportunities.

Discontinuation of Transmission-Based Precautions

Transmission-Based Precautions remain in effect for limited periods of time (i.e., while the risk for transmission of the infectious agent persists or for the duration of the illness. For some diseases (e.g., pharyngeal or cutaneous diphtheria, RSV), Transmission-Based Precautions remain in effect until culture or antigen-detection test results document eradication of the pathogen and, for RSV, symptomatic disease is resolved. For other diseases (e.g., *M. tuberculosis*), state laws and regulations, and health care facility policies, may dictate the duration of precautions. In immunocompromised patients, viral shedding can persist for prolonged periods of time (many weeks to months) and transmission to others may occur during that time; therefore, the duration of contact and/or droplet precautions may be prolonged for many weeks.

Application of Transmission-Based Precautions in Ambulatory and Home Care Settings

Although Transmission-Based Precautions generally apply in all health care settings, exceptions exist. For example, in home care, AIIRs are not available. Furthermore, family members already exposed to diseases such as varicella and tuberculosis would not use masks or respiratory protection, but visiting phlebotomists or other health care workers would need to use such protection. Similarly, management of patients colonized or infected with multidrug-resistant organisms may necessitate Contact Precautions in acute-care hospitals and in some long-term care facilities when there is continued transmission, but the risk of transmission in ambulatory care and home care has not been defined. Consistent use of Standard Precautions may suffice in these settings, but more information is needed.

Appendix C

Review of Body Systems

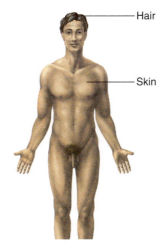

Integumentary System

Provides protection, regulates temperature, prevents water loss, and produces vitamin D precursors. Consists of skin, hair, nails, and sweat glands.

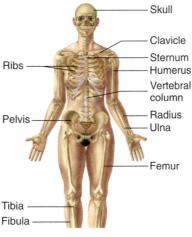

Skeletal System

Provides protection and support, allows body movements, produces blood cells, and stores minerals and fat. Consists of bones, associated cartilages, ligaments, and joints.

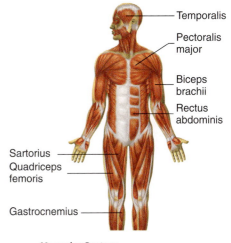

Muscular System

Produces body movements, maintains posture, and produces body heat. Consists of muscles attached to the skeleton by tendons.

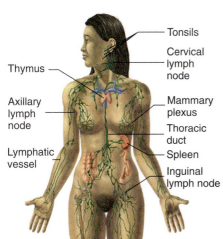

Lymphatic System

Removes foreign substances from the blood and lymph, combats disease, maintains tissue fluid balance, and absorbs fats from the digestive tract. Consists of the lymphatic vessels, lymph nodes, and other lymphatic organs.

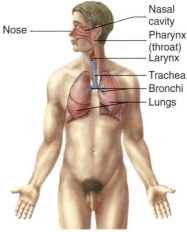

Respiratory System

Exchanges oxygen and carbon dioxide between the blood and air and regulates blood pH. Consists of the lungs and respiratory passages.

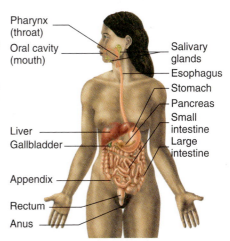

Digestive System

Performs the mechanical and chemical processes of digestion, absorption of nutrients, and elimination of wastes. Consists of the mouth, esophagus, stomach, intestines, and accessory organs.

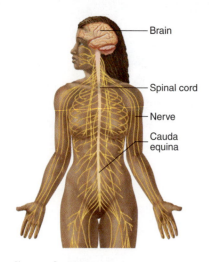

Nervous System

A major regulatory system that detects sensations and controls movements, physiologic processes, and intellectual functions. Consists of the brain, spinal cord, nerves, and sensory receptors.

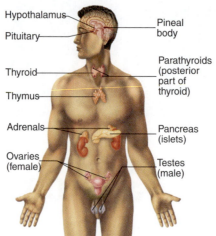

Endocrine System

A major regulatory system that influences metabolism, growth, reproduction, and many other functions. Consists of glands, such as the pituitary, that secrete hormones.

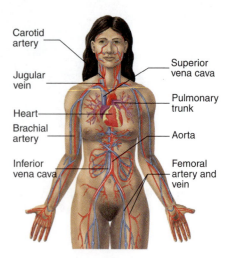

Cardiovascular System

Transports nutrients, waste products, gases, and hormones throughout the body; plays a role in the immune response and the regulation of body temperature. Consists of the heart, blood vessels, and blood.

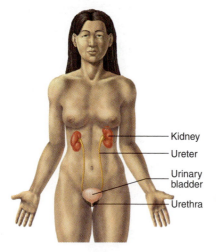

Urinary System

Removes waste products from the blood and regulates blood pH, ion balance, and water balance. Consists of the kidneys, urinary bladder, and ducts that carry urine.

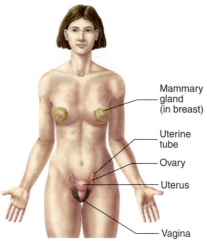

Female Reproductive System

Produces oocytes and is the site of fertilization and fetal development; produces milk for the newborn; produces hormones that influence sexual function and behaviors. Consists of the ovaries, vagina, uterus, mammary glands, and associated structures.

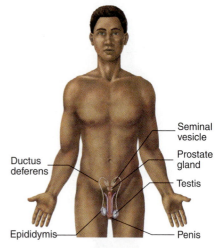

Male Reproductive System

Produces and transfers sperm cells to the female and produces hormones that influence sexual functions and behaviors. Consists of the testes, accessory structures, ducts, and penis.

Competency Checklists

Use these Competency Checklists in your classroom, laboratory, or clinical setting. During classroom training, you can review the procedures presented in the book in a step-by-step format. The competency checklists further divide each procedure into preprocedure, procedure, and postprocedure sections for simplicity and ease of review. For learning the hands-on procedures of phlebotomy, the checklist format provides a place to mark your practice and proficiency. In addition, there are areas for the instructor or clinical supervisor to document that you have mastered the competency. Completed Competency Checklists can be placed in your educational or employment portfolio.

Competency Checklist: Venipuncture Using an Evacuated Tube

Procedure Steps	Practice			Performed		Master
	1	2	3	Yes	No	
Preprocedure						
1. Examines requisition slip/form						
2. Greets the patient, introduces self						
3. Identifies patient verbally using two identifiers						
4. Examines patient's ID band						
5. Compares requisition form with ID band						
6. States procedure to be performed						
7. Verifies diet restrictions or instructions						
8. Puts on gloves						
9. Selects correct equipment and supplies						
10. Assembles correct equipment and supplies						
11. Conveniently places equipment						
12. Reassures patient						
13. Positions patient's arm						
14. Applies tourniquet						
15. Identifies a vein by palpation						
16. Selects venipuncture site						
17. Releases tourniquet						
18. Cleanses venipuncture site						
19. Allows site to air dry						
Procedure						
1. Reapplies tourniquet						
2. Confirms the venipuncture site visually						
3. Anchors vein below puncture site						
4. Smoothly inserts needle at correct angle						
5. Inserts needle with bevel up						

(Continued)

Procedure Steps	Practice			Performed		Master
	1	2	3	Yes	No	
Procedure						
6. Inserts tubes without causing pain						
7. Allows tubes to fill completely						
8. Removes tubes						
9. Mixes tubes by inversion						
10. Collects tubes in correct order						
11. Does not move needle between tubes						
12. Removes last tube from holder						
13. Releases the tourniquet						
14. Places gauze over puncture site						
15. Withdraws the needle smoothly						
Postprocedure						
1. Applies pressure to venipuncture site						
2. Disposes of needle and tube adaptor in correct container						
3. Labels tubes correctly						
4. Observes special handling instructions						
5. Checks the patient's arm						
6. Applies bandage						
7. Thanks the patient						
8. Disposes of used supplies appropriately						
9. Removes gloves and washes hands						
10. Transports specimens to the laboratory						

Comments: _____

_____

_____

_____

Signed

Evaluator: _____

Student: _____

Competency Checklist: Venipuncture Using a Syringe

Procedure Steps	Practice			Performed		Master
	1	2	3	Yes	No	
Preprocedure						
1. Examines requisition slip/form						
2. Greets the patient, introduces self						
3. Identifies patient verbally using two identifiers						
4. Examines patient's ID band						
5. Compares requisition form with ID band						
6. States procedure to be performed						
7. Verifies diet restrictions or instructions						
8. Puts on gloves						
9. Selects correct equipment and supplies						
10. Assembles correct equipment and supplies						
11. Checks plunger movement of syringe						
12. Conveniently places equipment						
13. Reassures patient						
14. Positions patient's arm						
15. Applies tourniquet						
16. Identifies a vein by palpation						
17. Selects venipuncture site						
18. Releases tourniquet						
19. Cleanses the venipuncture site						
20. Allows site to air dry						
Procedure						
1. Reapplies tourniquet						
2. Confirms the venipuncture site visually						
3. Anchors vein below puncture site						

(Continued)

Procedure Steps	Practice			Performed		Master
	1	2	3	Yes	No	
Procedure						
4. Smoothly inserts needle at correct angle						
5. Inserts needle with bevel up						
6. Collects appropriate amount of sample						
7. Releases the tourniquet						
8. Places gauze over puncture site						
9. Withdraws the needle smoothly						
Postprocedure						
1. Applies pressure to venipuncture site						
2. Uses safe technique to fill tubes						
3. Fills tubes in correct order						
4. Mixes anticoagulated tubes by inversion						
5. Disposes of needle in correct container						
6. Disposes of syringe correctly						
7. Labels tubes correctly						
8. Observes special handling instructions						
9. Checks the patient's arm						
10. Applies bandage						
11. Thanks the patient						
12. Disposes of used supplies appropriately						
13. Removes gloves and washes hands						
14. Transports specimens to the laboratory						

Comments: _____

_____

_____

_____

Signed

Evaluator: _____

Student: _____

Name: _____ Date: _____

Competency Checklist: Transferring Specimen to Tubes

Procedure Steps	Practice			Performed		Master
	1	2	3	Yes	No	
Preprocedure						
1. Starts specimen transfer procedure immediately after removing needle from arm						
2. Selects correct equipment and supplies						
3. Uses blood transfer device						
4. Conveniently places equipment						
Procedure						
1. Inserts syringe into transfer device hub						
2. Transfers the specimen into tubes						
3. Uses safe technique to fill tubes						
4. Fills tubes in correct order						
5. Allows tubes to fill naturally						
6. Mixes anticoagulated tubes by inversion						
Postprocedure						
1. Disposes of transfer device and syringe in correct container						
2. Labels tubes correctly						
3. Observes special handling instructions						
4. Disposes of used supplies appropriately						
5. Removes gloves and washes hands						
6. Transports specimens to the laboratory						

Comments: _____

_____

_____

_____

Signed

Evaluator: _____

Student: _____

Competency Checklist: Dermal Puncture on Finger

Procedure Steps	Practice			Performed		Master
	1	2	3	Yes	No	
Preprocedure						
1. Examines requisition slip/form						
2. Greets the patient, introduces self						
3. Identifies patient verbally using two identifiers						
4. Examines patient's ID band						
5. Compares requisition form with ID band						
6. States procedure to be performed						
7. Verifies diet restrictions or instructions						
8. Puts on gloves						
9. Selects correct equipment and supplies						
10. Assembles correct equipment and supplies						
11. Conveniently places equipment						
12. Reassures patient						
13. Selects appropriate finger						
14. Warms finger if necessary						
15. Selects dermal puncture site						
16. Cleanses the puncture site						
17. Allows site to air dry						
Procedure						
1. Ensures that unclean finger does not touch site						
2. Does not contaminate puncture device						
3. Performs puncture smoothly						
4. Punctures appropriate site across fingerprint						
5. Wipes away first drop of blood						
6. Collects rounded drops of blood						

(Continued)

Procedure Steps	Practice			Performed		Master
	1	2	3	Yes	No	
Procedure						
7. Collects sample without scraping						
8. Collects without milking site						
9. Collects appropriate amount of sample						
10. Mixes Microtainer® or seals tubes						
11. Cleanses site						
12. Places gauze over puncture site						
Postprocedure						
1. Applies pressure to puncture site						
2. Removes all items from collection area						
3. Disposes of puncture device correctly						
4. Labels tubes correctly						
5. Observes special handling instructions						
6. Checks the patient's finger						
7. Applies bandage						
8. Thanks the patient						
9. Disposes of used supplies appropriately						
10. Removes gloves and washes hands						
11. Transports specimens to the laboratory						

Comments: _____

_____

_____

_____

Signed

Evaluator: _____

Student: _____

Name: _____   Date: _____

Competency Checklist: Dermal Puncture on Heel

Procedure Steps	Practice 1	Practice 2	Practice 3	Performed Yes	Performed No	Master
Preprocedure						
1. Examines requisition slip/form						
2. Greets the patient and parents						
3. Places collection tray in appropriate area						
4. Examines patient's ID band						
5. Compares requisition form with ID band using two identifiers						
6. States procedure to parents						
7. Puts on gloves						
8. Selects correct equipment and supplies						
9. Assembles correct equipment and supplies						
10. Conveniently places equipment						
11. Reassures patient and parents						
12. Warms heel area if necessary						
13. Selects dermal puncture site on heel						
14. Cleanses the puncture site						
15. Allows site to air dry						
Procedure						
1. Ensures that unclean finger does not touch site						
2. Does not contaminate puncture device						
3. Performs puncture smoothly						
4. Punctures appropriate site						
5. Wipes away first drop of blood						
6. Collects rounded drops of blood						
7. Collects sample without scraping						
8. Collects without milking site						

(Continued)

Procedure Steps	Practice			Performed		Master
	1	2	3	Yes	No	
Procedure						
9. Collects appropriate amount of sample						
10. Mixes Microtainer® or seals tubes						
11. Cleanses site						
12. Places gauze over puncture site						
Postprocedure						
1. Applies pressure to puncture site						
2. Applies pressure until bleeding stops						
3. Removes all items from collection area						
4. Disposes of puncture device correctly						
5. Labels tubes correctly						
6. Observes special handling instructions						
7. Checks the patient's heel						
8. Applies bandage (optional)						
9. Thanks the patient and parents						
10. Disposes of used supplies appropriately						
11. Removes gloves and washes hands						
12. Transports specimens to the laboratory						

Comments: _____

_____

_____

_____

Signed

Evaluator: _____

Student: _____

Name: _____ Date: _____

Competency Checklist: Centrifuge Operation

Procedure Steps	Practice 1	2	3	Performed Yes	No	Master
Preprocedure						
1. Puts on gloves						
2. Transports specimen to centrifuge area						
3. Conveniently places specimens						
4. Opens lid of centrifuge						
Procedure						
1. Inserts tubes so that they are balanced						
2. Does not remove caps from tubes						
3. If cap is missing, covers end of tube						
4. Closes centrifuge lid						
5. Locks lid into place						
6. Sets centrifuge time and speed correctly						
Postprocedure						
1. Allows centrifuge to stop completely						
2. Opens lid after centrifuge has stopped						
3. Observes special handling instructions						
4. If tubes are broken, cleans appropriately						
5. Disposes of used supplies appropriately						
6. Removes gloves and washes hands						

Comments: _____

_____

_____

_____

Signed

Evaluator: _____

Student: _____

Name: _____   Date: _____

Competency Checklist: Venipuncture Using a Butterfly and Syringe or Adaptor

Procedure Steps	Practice			Performed		Master
	1	2	3	Yes	No	
Preprocedure						
1. Examines requisition slip/form						
2. Greets the patient, introduces self						
3. Identifies patient verbally using two identifiers						
4. Examines patient's ID band						
5. Compares requisition form with ID band						
6. States procedure to be performed						
7. Verifies diet restrictions or instructions						
8. Puts on gloves						
9. Selects correct equipment and supplies						
10. Assembles correct equipment and supplies						
11. Checks plunger movement of syringe						
12. Or checks tube adaptor						
13. Conveniently places equipment						
14. Reassures patient, positions patient's arm						
15. Applies tourniquet						
16. Identifies a vein by palpation						
17. Selects a venipuncture site						
18. Releases tourniquet						
19. Cleanses the venipuncture site						
20. Allows site to air dry						
Procedure						
1. Reapplies tourniquet						
2. Confirms the venipuncture site visually						
3. Anchors vein below puncture site						
4. Holds butterfly needle by the wings						

(Continued)

Procedure Steps	Practice			Performed		Master
	1	2	3	Yes	No	
Procedure						
5. Smoothly inserts needle at correct angle						
6. Inserts needle with bevel up						
7. Collects appropriate amount of sample						
8. Or fills tubes in correct order (adaptor)						
9. Mixes anticoagulated tubes by inversion						
10. Releases the tourniquet						
11. Places gauze over puncture site						
12. Withdraws the needle smoothly						
Postprocedure						
1. Applies pressure to venipuncture site						
2. Uses safe technique to fill tubes (syringe)						
3. Fills tubes in correct order (syringe)						
4. Mixes anticoagulated tubes by inversion						
5. Disposes of butterfly in correct container						
6. Disposes of syringe in correct container						
7. Labels tubes correctly						
8. Observes special handling instructions						
9. Checks the patient's arm						
10. Disposes of used supplies apropriately						
11. Removes gloves and washes hands						
12. Transports specimens to the laboratory						

Comments: _____

_____

_____

_____

Signed

Evaluator: _____

Student: _____

Appendix E

Answer Key

Chapter One

Checkpoint Question 1-1

1. Obtain blood specimens either by venipuncture or dermal puncture, remove blood from donors, collect and package urine, accept and route specimens to the correct department for testing and analysis.

Checkpoint Question 1-2

1. It was believed to rid the body of impurities, evil spirits, unwanted diseases, and fever.

Troubleshooting: Providing Customer Service

1. As you call each patient back into the laboratory, you should be professional. Use a calm tone to explain the situation and tell the patient you are very sorry for the delay. Ignoring the situation could cause the patients to become more upset.

Checkpoint Questions 1-3

1. See Table 1-1.
2. In a calm voice, apologize to the patient for the delay and explain the reason in a professional manner.

Checkpoint Questions 1-4

1. A waived test has much less risk to the patient as determined by the Clinical Laboratory Improvement Act. They are most commonly performed in a physician's office laboratory and involve small amounts of blood or other easily obtainable specimen.
2. Microbiology—the study of microscopic organisms
   Chemistry—evaluation of chemical constituents of the human body

Hematology—study of blood and blood-forming tissues
Immunology—the study of the body's resistance to disease
Serology—the identification of antibodies in the blood's serum
Urinalysis—examination of the urine
Toxicology—detection and study of the adverse effects of chemicals on living organisms
Blood banking—the area of the lab for donated blood including type and cross-match and blood processing

Checkpoint Questions 1-5

1. CLIA '88
2. JCAHO

Checkpoint Questions 1-6

1. Perform hand hygiene, follow Standard Precautions, wear personal protective equipment.
2. Apply—gown, mask or respirator, goggles or face shield, then gloves
   Remove—gloves, face shield or goggles, gown, then mask or respirator

Checkpoint Questions 1-7

1. Any three of the following:
   Close patients' room doors when caring for them or discussing their health.
   Do not talk about patients in public places.
   Turn computer screens that contain patient information so passersby cannot see the information.

Log off computers when you are done.

Do not walk away from patient medical records; close them when leaving.

2. You should discuss the results of your test with the physician or other licensed practitioner. I am not allowed to disclose or discuss results with you.

Chapter Review

Multiple Choice

1. b	5. d	8. b
2. a	6. b	9. d
3. d	7. d	10. a
4. c		

Fill in the Blanks

11. Verbal = using slang or street language; using medical terminology

    Nonverbal = improper grooming or attire; avoiding eye contact; not respecting personal space

12. Inpatient settings = hospitals; rehabilitation centers; nursing homes

    Outpatient settings = American Red Cross; physician offices; ambulatory care centers

13. Point-of-care testing

True or False

14. True
15. False—Members of the health care team may be trained to perform phlebotomy, such as physicians, nurses, medical assistants, paramedics, and patient care assistants.
16. False—Venipuncture requires the use of a sharp object that is introduced into a vein, and a larger blood sample is obtained than with a dermal puncture.
17. True
18. True
19. True
20. False—Venipuncture is used for larger blood samples.

Matching Game

21. d	23. a	25. c
22. e	24. b	

What Should You Do?

26. No, the phlebotomist should go to the nurse caring for the patient, or a family member who can speak English. All patients are legally entitled to give their consent for procedures, and hospitals receiving funding from the Department of Health and Human Services must provide an interpreter if no family is available.

27. The phlebotomist should politely request the visitors to wait outside for a moment while the patient's blood is obtained and should inform the inquisitive visitor that the phlebotomist cannot provide information about tests or results ordered by the physician.

28. Initially, using a very soft, easy tone and mannerisms, the phlebotomist should remind the patient that the physician ordered the tests to assist with evaluating the patient's condition. If the patient continues to refuse, the phlebotomist should leave as requested, document the incident thoroughly, and notify the physician.

29. The phlebotomist believed that because it wasn't her fault that the patient had to wait, it wasn't her place to deal with the patient's frustration about it. However, the patients are the customers and should be treated with good customer service. The phlebotomist should have addressed the problem with each patient briefly, explaining what had occurred without acting irritated or upset. Addressing the problem and helping the patients understand will reduce their frustration, thus providing improved customer service and fewer patient complaints.

30. You should remind the co-worker that equipment should not leave the room of a patient in isolation because of the chance of contamination. All equipment on the tray must be left in the room and/or the proper cleaning procedure must be implemented. If the tray is taken into another patient's room there is a chance that patient will become contaminated.

Chapter Two

Checkpoint Question 2-1

1. Cellular and liquid components of blood, closed circuit of blood vessels, location of blood vessels, and composition of blood.

Checkpoint Question 2-2

1. Coronary—blood travels to and from the heart to maintain the muscular pump. Pulmonary—blood travels to and from the lungs to remove carbon dioxide and

obtain oxygen. Systemic—blood travels to and from the body through the heart for exchange of oxygen, carbon dioxide, nutrients, and waste.

Troubleshooting: Artery or Vein?

1. Remove the needle, apply firm pressure for at least five minutes, apply a taut gauze dressing, and instruct the patient to keep the arm still for a short period of time.

Checkpoint Questions 2-3

1. Aorta (largest artery)—arteries—arterioles—capillaries—venules—veins—superior or inferior vena cava (vein)
2. median cubital, cephalic, and basilic

Checkpoint Questions 2-4

1. Red blood cells carry hemoglobin. Hemoglobin provides the ability for red blood cells to transport oxygen and carbon dioxide.
2. Destroying foreign substances and removing cellular debris
3. Serum is the liquid portion of blood that has been allowed to clot in a tube. Plasma is the liquid portion of blood that has not clotted and has been centrifuged.

Troubleshooting: Lack of Clotting Factors

1. Hold firm pressure with the gauze for at least three to five minutes.

Checkpoint Question 2-5

1. blood vessel spasm—platelet plug formation—blood clotting—fibrinolysis

Troubleshooting: Blood Suppliers

1. 17 years old, good health, and over 110 pounds

Checkpoint Questions 2-6

1. Identify the patient with two identifiers and label all blood and blood products completely and accurately.
2. To ensure that the blood given to a patient does not cause a transfusion reaction

Chapter Review

Label the Figure

1. a   3. b   4. a
2. c

Matching

5. d   11. h   17. p
6. j   12. e   18. k
7. l   13. f   19. a
8. n   14. o   20. g
9. b   15. i
10. c   16. m

True or False

21. False. Only veins have valves to prevent the backflow of blood.
22. True
23. True
24. True
25. True
26. False. There are 70,000 miles of blood vessels in the vascular system.
27. False. Capillaries are the smallest of the vessel family, and their primary function is to provide a link between arterioles and venules and allow the transfer of gases and other substances between the blood and other body cells.
28. False. Pulmonary circulation consists of oxygenated blood leaving the lungs and heading back to the heart to be pumped into all the body systems.
29. True
30. True

Matching

31. h   34. i   37. c
32. f   35. g   38. e
33. d   36. a   39. b

Ordering

40. 2   42. 3   43. 4
41. 1

Fill in the Blanks

44. Antigens
45. Serum
46. Antibodies
47. A
48. O

What Should You Do?

49. Accidental arterial puncture; remove the needle and apply firm pressure for at least five minutes, notify the nurse, and ask patient to keep arm still once a firm dressing is applied.

50. Come back at a later time when the phlebotomist would have time to apply personal protective equipment and perform good handwashing. This patient already has a low resistance to infection, so proper time is required for handwashing and PPE needs to be worn.
51. Eosinophils
52. T-lymphocytes and B-lymphocytes
53. A patient with low platelets would be prone to bleeding. When collecting blood you should apply pressure for a minimum of three to five minutes to make sure the bleeding stops at the site.

Get Connected

1. Students can search any of the materials available on this site and find multiple pictures to print and create a bulletin board or develop a presentation.

Chapter Three

Checkpoint Question 3-1

1. The equipment, ordering process, and paper or computer work necessary prior to collection.

Troubleshooting: Patient Identification

Verify the correct spelling of the name and compare the information with at least one other identifier such as the date of birth or medical record number.

Checkpoint Questions 3-2

1. Patient name, ordering physician's name, medical record number, date and time test performed, type of test, test status, patient location, Social Security number, and date of birth.
2. Receive orders, print requisitions, maintain patient data, add patient charges, and keep patient test results.

Troubleshooting: Hemolysis

The blood will need to be re-collected using a needle and tube that match in size.

Checkpoint Questions 3-3

1. Gloves, tourniquet, alcohol prep pads, gauze pads, adhesive bandage or tape, needles, evacuated tube holder or syringe, sharps container, permanent marker, computer label, or pen, evacuated tubes.

2. Tubes are color coded and have no additives or various additives that react with the blood to make it suitable for the test that is being performed. Selection is based on the type of specimen needed and test ordered. For example, an anticoagulant is used to prevent the blood from clotting when plasma is needed for the blood test.
3. Hemoglobin A1C should be a lavender tube. Cholesterol should be an SST tube. The SST tube should be filled first.

Checkpoint Questions 3-4

1. Infants and children under two, adults with veins that are difficult to stick due to burns, chemotherapy patients, elderly patients, and patients performing home glucose monitoring.
2. Red-tipped tubes that are coated with heparin to prevent clotting, blue tipped tubes that do not contain heparin, and black-tipped tubes that are used for smaller quantities of blood.

Chapter Review

True or False

1. True
2. True
3. True
4. False. A bacteriostatic antiseptic inhibits the growth of bacteria
5. True
6. False. Yellow-topped tubes contain sodium polyanethol sulfonate (SPS) or acid citrate dextrose (ACD).
7. False. Sharps containers are bright orange and must be made of a nonpenetrable material such as plastic. Soft plastic is not used.
8. True

Labeling

9. Evacuated tube
10. Flange
11. Rubber stopper on tube
12. Evacuated tube holder
13. Needle

Matching

14. f	17. c	19. b
15. g	18. a	20. d
16. e		

Fill in the Blanks

21. Light blue
22. Red
23. Lavender
24. Gray
25. Green

Ordering

26. 2	**29.** 6	**32.** 5
27. 1	**30.** 3	**33.** 8
28. 7	**31.** 4	

Multiple Choice

34. b	**37.** d	**40.** b
35. c	**38.** c	**41.** a
36. d	**39.** a	**42.** a

What Should You Do?

43. Discard the damaged needle because it could cause injury to the patient or inhibit the blood collection process. Open another needle for the venipuncture.

44. Use capillary or microspecimen collection procedures because it is easier to collect blood from an infant by dermal puncture. It is less traumatic for the infant, and usually enough blood can be collected by dermal puncture.

45. If you or your patient is allergic, avoid all items that contain latex including gloves, tourniquets, bandages, and tape. Always ask the patient if he or she is allergic to latex.

46. **(a)** CBC is lavender-topped tube, PT and PTT use a light blue-topped tube. The light blue tube should be drawn first. If using a butterfly set, a red-topped tube should be used and discarded.

    (b) Either a red tube or an SST (red-gray) tube can be used for both cholesterol and triglycerides. Check the facility policy.

    (c) Blood culture is first using blood culture yellow-topped tube; potassium is next, using a SST red-gray or gold-topped tube; and gray-topped tube is drawn last for the alcohol level.

Get Connected *Internet Activity*

1. This link will provide the latest regulations for safe-needle standards, including pictures, PowerPoint presentations, and other materials that can be used for the students' summary.

The following is an example of information provided at the site. Most importantly the summary should provide all the guideline as follows: As of 2001 the Needlestick Safety and Prevention Act mandated the use of safe-needle devices and required that health care facilities use alternatives to needles where possible and use devices with safety features when a needle is required. Because of the Needlestick Safety and Prevention Act, health care facilities are now required to:

- Document the evaluation and implementation of safety-engineered sharp devices and needleless systems.
- Review and update exposure control plans at least annually to reflect changes in sharps safety technology.
- Maintain a sharps injury log.
- Include frontline health care workers (actual users of the equipment) in the evaluation and selection process of safety-engineered sharp devices.
- Expand of the definition of "engineering controls" to include devices with engineered sharps injury protection. These controls (e.g., sharps disposal containers, self-sheathing needles, and needleless systems) should isolate or remove the bloodborne pathogens hazard from the workplace.

Employers are obligated to provide the equipment and controls to reduce the possibility of needlestick injuries, and employees have the responsibility to protect themselves and co-workers from needlestick injuries by doing the following:

- Avoid the use of needles when possible.
- Correctly use the safe alternatives provided.
- Don't recap needles.
- Dispose of used needles promptly and in an appropriate sharps container.
- Report hazards from needles you observe in the workplace.
- Report needlestick injuries promptly to ensure you receive appropriate follow-up care.
- Attend training and follow infection control policies and procedures.

Most needlestick injuries occur during or after use and before disposal of the needle. They are usually related to recapping and failing to dispose of used needles properly. Safe-needle devices are designed to decrease risks during all aspects of IV therapy. There are many types of safe-needle devices in use. Ideally, devices should

- be needleless
- be built into the device
- require no activation by the user (a passive device) or, if user activation is necessary, the safety feature can be activated without exposing the user to the sharp point and easily enables the user to tell that it is activated
- be easy to use and practical
- be safe and effective for patient care.

2. The student will find multiple resources for phlebotomy equipment and education here. There are wall charts and tube charts that are kept up to date with the current standards. The final project should reflect the latest information, including pictures of various tubes for phlebotomy.

Chapter Four

Checkpoint Question 4-1

1. Using aseptic technique, following standard precautions, obtaining the correct specimen from the correct patient.

Troubleshooting: Wake the Patient Gently

1. Nudge the bed, rather than the patient. Talk softly and avoid turning on the bright lights.

Troubleshooting: Patient Refusal

"Refused," date, time, initials, and name of licensed practitioner informed of refusal.

Troubleshooting: Petechiae

Caused by tourniquet on too long. Remove the tourniquet in a timely manner (one minute or less).

Troubleshooting: Hematoma

Apply pressure and ice to the site.

Troubleshooting: Hemoconcentration

The patient should not pump the fist. You should not place the tourniquet on too tight or for longer than one minute.

Troubleshooting: Use of Alcohol

To prevent burning sensation and a hemoplyzed specimen. Also to dry out the bacteria.

Checkpoint Questions 4-2

1. Assembling the equipment, greeting the patient, identifying the patient and explaining the procedure, verifying dietary restrictions, positioning the patient, applying the tourniquet, selecting the venipuncture site, and cleansing the venipuncture site.
2. Children, geriatric patients, patients with HIV or hepatitis, mentally ill patients, patients with IV, mastectomy, and/or lymphostasis

Troubleshooting: Handling Syncope

Remove the tourniquet and needle while calling for help. Apply pressure to venipuncture site and stand in front of the patient to prevent him/her from falling.

Checkpoint Questions 4-3

1. You see blood in the evacuated tube after the tube is completely inserted.
2. An overfilled evacuated tube is less likely because the vacuum in the tube will only draw blood into the tube while the vacuum is present and the filling will stop. A tube can be underfilled if the phlebotomist removes it from the needle before vacuum is gone.

Checkpoint Questions 4-4

1. Engage the safety mechanism—the timing will depend upon the type of safety needle being used.
2. After the blood is in the tube and before you leave the patient.

Checkpoint Questions 4-5

1. A butterfly needle set should only be used as a last resort because of the increased potential for accidental needlesticks.
2. A safety blood transfer device is used to prevent accidental needlesticks.

Troubleshooting: Crying Infant

Wait at least 60 minutes after the procedure to prevent an elevated leukocyte count.

Checkpoint Questions 4-6

1. A newborn would most likely have a dermal puncture. A 10-month-old infant may be walking so a dermal is not desirable. An elderly may have a dermal puncture; however, it is best to use a venipuncture unless a specimen cannot be obtained by venipuncture.

2. The site for the puncture and the type of equipment are the two main differences between dermal puncture and venipuncture.

Chapter Review

Multiple Choice

1. d	8. b	15. d
2. d	9. a	16. c
3. d	10. b	17. a
4. c	11. b	18. c
5. c	12. a	19. a
6. b	13. c	
7. d	14. c	

Ordering

20. k, g, d, c, b, h, f, l, j, a, m, i, e

Matching

21. a	25. g	29. j
22. c	26. h	30. i
23. d	27. f	
24. b	28. e	

True or False

31. True
32. False. STAT tests are usually obtained before your routine specimens.
33. False. Vacutainer® tubes must be filled completely to ensure accurate testing.
34. False. Never unscrew the needle from the adaptor. Dispose of the needle and adaptor together.
35. True

What Should You Do?

36. Concerns could include the following: With children present, the venipuncture could frighten them or could make them very curious and want to watch closely. The adults present may judge your ability to handle the situation and/or procedure. You need to provide privacy for the patient. You nicely ask Mr. Tykodi to go back to his room with you. It may be nice and sunny in the waiting area, but you cannot control the surrounding area and people. Other people in the room may not react well to seeing blood drawn, and his grandson may not react well either. It probably is a good idea to have Mr. Tykodi lie down as his blood is being taken in case he begins to not feel well.

37. You go out to the pediatric floor nurses' station for help. Ask if someone (possibly the nurse in charge of Jennifer) could assist you in the blood collection for Jennifer Burnham. You should not attempt to draw Jennifer's blood by yourself. She is already upset about the procedure and may become even more difficult. Try to talk to her in a kind, calm manner and ask her to help in the collection procedure. Tell her you will give her a special bandage if she helps.

38. You should verify the patient information with complete accuracy. Double-check with the requisition, patient chart, and/or the attending nurse regarding the discrepancy. Do not draw the blood unless the names are exactly the same. Even a one letter or number difference is not acceptable for phlebotomy.

39. This specimen should not be used. No guessing allowed. Discard the specimen. Carefully check each patient's requisition and tubes obtained. Try to determine which patient may be missing a specimen. Report this to your supervisor or the physician to determine if another order or specimen must be obtained.

40. You must keep your number of attempts to two. Do not try to stick the patient again. Report to your supervisor or follow the protocol at the facility where you are working. In some cases, you may ask a co-worker to draw the blood. Remain calm so as not to upset the patient further.

Get Connected

1. The table should include the common complications such as ecchymosis, petechiae,

hemoconcentration, pain, hematoma, and syncope. A complete table will include proper procedure for handling each situation. In a class or group discussion, compare tables and/or make one complete table with all the information collected to use during externship.

Chapter Five

Checkpoint Question 5-1

1. Perform special handling or processing procedures, collect other specimens, and perform some tests immediately at the point of care.

Checkpoint Questions 5-2

1. Answers will vary. Three critical steps to perform during blood culture include: avoid false positives by using proper technique to avoid contaminants, avoid false negatives by collecting enough blood, collect more than one set of blood cultures at two different sites or at two different times at least 45 minutes apart.
2. Answers will vary. Examples of tests that require the following special handling: heat—cold agglutinins; ice-water mixture—arterial blood gases; darkness—bilirubin.

Troubleshooting: Unopettes®

The reagent in the reservoir is designed for a specific amount of blood. If the amount of blood is wrong, the results will be wrong.

Checkpoint Question 5-3

1. The Unopette® is a microcollection device. The two parts are a reservoir and a pipette.

Checkpoint Questions 5-4

1. The tube should remain in the source of blood or horizontal during the filling process.
2. The tube is kept horizontal and sealed as required.

Checkpoint Question 5-5

1. Answers will vary. Any three criteria as identified in Table 5-1.

Checkpoint Questions 5-6

1. Point-of-care blood tests include glucose, hemoglobin, sodium, potassium, chloride, bicarbonate, ionized, calcium, cholesterol, blood ketones, blood gases, hemoglobin A1C, and coagulation studies such as prothrombin time (PT), activated partial thromboplastin time (APTT), and activated clotting time.
2. POCT is designed to reduce health care cost, provide immediate feedback for patients to improve compliance and health care personnel to provide quick diagnosis and treatment.

Checkpoint Questions 5-7

1. A test must be completed on a urine specimen within an hour or the specimen should be refrigerated.
2. A reagent strip has a chemical reagent on a plastic strip used to dip into a urine specimen to test for the presence and concentration of various substances.

Checkpoint Question 5-8

1. Glucose, potassium, and coagulation studies are most affected by improper centrifuging or centrifuging not done within the expected time limit of two hours after collection.

Chapter Review

Multiple Choice

1. d	6. a	11. c
2. c	7. a	12. c
3. d	8. b	13. b
4. d	9. c	14. a
5. c	10. b	15. b

True or False

16. True
17. True
18. False. The most common type of POCT is blood glucose.
19. False. If urine is kept at room temperature for more than one hour it can alter the test results of your chemical and microscopic components.
20. True

Matching

21. i	25. b	29. j
22. f	26. h	30. d
23. a	27. e	
24. g	28. c	

What Should You Do?

31. It does not matter who drew the specimen or who dropped it off in the processing area.

You should report to the physician who ordered the test that it just came into the laboratory and the results will possibly be erroneous due to the age of the specimen and another specimen should be drawn.

32. Put the collected specimen immediately on ice, then go back to the laboratory and see if the 10-minute delay is critical. Most likely, you will have to recollect the specimen from Mrs. Diaz.

33. Because you are not certain you did the proper cleaning, the test could result in a false positive. Also, a second site should be used for the second set of blood culture tubes. If these procedures were not performed, you will need to complete the test again, making sure you cleaned the area completely and properly and collected the correct number of containers of blood from two different sites or at two different times at least 45 minutes apart.

Get Connected

1. Six factors that influence the quality of the specimen and prevent pre-analytical errors are the right specimen, right collection, right labeling, right quantity, right transport, and right storage.

Chapter Six

Checkpoint Question 6-1

1. Patient behaviors that can affect test results include exercise, eating, posture, stress, smoking, and drinking alcohol.

Checkpoint Questions 6-2

1. Fasting should be for 8 to 12 hours.
2. The blood test most affected by non-fasting are glucose and triglycerides.

Checkpoint Questions 6-3

1. During a glucose tolerance test the patient can pass out and fall. A patient can also become nauseated and vomit or may sneak a snack that can affect the results of the test.
2. A one-hour glucose challenge screening test is done on a patient who is at risk for gestational diabetes.

Troubleshooting: Notify the Physician

coumadin, heparin, warfarin, aspirin, and aspirin-containing medications

Checkpoint Question 6-4

1. The platelet function assay is replacing the bleeding time test because it is less invasive and the bleeding time test is not sensitive to patients who are taking non-steroidal anti-inflammatory agents and aspirin products.

Checkpoint Questions 6-5

1. Therapeutic blood collection is done to treat such diseases as polycythemia and hemachromatosis. Autologous blood donation is done by a patient so he or she will have blood available for a future surgical procedure.
2. Patients should be made aware of the need for a safe blood supply so they will answer questions honestly about behaviors that can place recipients of their blood at risk.

Checkpoint Questions 6-6

1. You should ensure that there is a legal document such as a court order before collecting a specimen for blood alcohol on a person with a possible DUI.
2. When collecting a forensic specimen you should wear gloves, collect as soon as possible, ensure proper storage (refrigerate for liquids) and packaging, labeling with the name, date of birth, your name, specimen type, and date and time of collection. Record collection and all handling on the appropriate document.

Checkpoint Questions 6-7

1. A peak drug level is drawn when the drug is at its highest level in the bloodstream, usually 15 to 30 minutes after the drug was administered.
2. A trough drug level is drawn when the drug is expected to be at its lowest concentration, usually immediately before administration of the next scheduled dose.

Checkpoint Question 6-8

1. Alternative sites used to obtain blood specimens include a heparin lock, central venous therapy line, arterial venous shunts, and an artery.

Chapter Review

Multiple Choice

1. d	6. c	12. b
2. c	7. b	12. c
3. c	8. d	13. d
4. d	9. a	14. d
5. c	10. a	15. b

Matching

16. j	21. a	26. b
17. k	22. c	27. d
18. i	23. e	28. f
19. g	24. o	29. h
20. l	25. m	30. n

True or False

31. False. A physician's order is required for autologous donation.
32. True
33. True
34. True
35. False. Autologous blood is blood donated by an individual for his or her future use.
36. False. Timed specimens are necessary for blood tests such as glucose and triglycerides.
37. False. Glucose levels aid in the diagnosis of diabetes.
38. True
39. False. Polycythemia is a disease that causes overproduction in the number of red blood cells.
40. True

What Should You Do?

41. Have the patient come back or wait ½ hour before you draw the blood. If the patient does not comply, you should notify the licensed practitioner who ordered the test.
42. You should not perform an arterial blood gas on your first official day as a phlebotomist. To obtain a blood specimen an arterial puncture is required, and to do this procedure you should have additional training or a special license, depending upon your facility and state of employment. You should politely explain that you do not feel qualified to draw an arterial blood gas and request another assignment.

Get Connected

1. Items on the list should include any or all of the following: fever, travel out of the country in the last 12 months, not feeling well, under the age of 17 or over the age of 66, less than 110 pounds, low hemoglobin or hematocrit, previous diagnosis or possible exposure to HIV, syphilis, or hepatitis.

Chapter Seven

Checkpoint Question 7-1

1. As a phlebotomist you should have knowledge of certification, continuing education, quality assurance, quality control, and risk management.

Checkpoint Questions 7-2

1. Certification is the process that ensures successful completion of defined academic and training requirements and a passing score on a national examination. Accreditation is the evaluation of the program of study, not the individual.
2. Continuing education can be obtained online, through staff development, workshops, and seminars.

Checkpoint Question 7-3

1. Other than laboratory results, patients would evaluate the care they received by how long they had to wait for the procedure, the presence or absence of bruising at the site, how many attempts, and their perception of the phlebotomist.

Troubleshooting: Using Quality Assurance Resources

The laboratory policy and procedure manual

Checkpoint Questions 7-4

1. Three quality control activities include calibration of equipment, validation of results, and documentation.
2. Answers will vary: The following are factors that can affect laboratory values—prolonged tourniquet placement, dietary state of patient not correct for test performed, incorrect volume of blood, order of the draw done incorrectly, proper handling of specimen (for example, some specimens must be chilled or protected from light).

Troubleshooting: Exposure Incident

Answers will vary: Not wearing gloves or accidental needlestick.

Checkpoint Questions 7-5

1. Malpractice is incorrect treatment of a patient. Negligence is failure to perform in a reasonable manner.
2. Answers will vary. See Table 7-1.
3. A material safety data sheet would be used to identify hazards of chemicals used and determine how accidental spills should be cleaned.

Chapter Review

Matching

1. g	4. c	7. e
2. d	5. h	8. f
3. b	6. a	

True or False

9. False. Customer satisfaction is the result of both the health care encounter and the accuracy of the results.
10. True
11. True
12. True
13. False. Clinical indicators are established during the assessment of the process.
14. False. A gray-topped tube is not full and might cause hemolysis and will be rejected.
15. True

Fill in the Blanks

16. Clinical Laboratory Standards Institute (CLIA)
17. Malpractice
18. OSHA Hazardous Communication Standard
19. CDC and OSHA
20. Scope of practice

Multiple Choice

21. d	23. b	25. b
22. b	24. c	

What Should You Do?

26. The phlebotomist should notify the nurse caring for the patient, or the physician, depending on the work setting, because this type of specimen should be drawn at the same time of day to ensure accurate results. The physician will probably reschedule the test. If this test is drawn without notifying the physician, it could give false results and lead to the wrong treatment.
27. The high control check reading indicates that the machine is out of the normal range. This machine would be considered inoperable until all the controls are within normal limits. The high control obtained does not meet precalibrated values. You should not use the machine. The use of defective equipment can alter the patient's treatments and lead to increased length of stay for the patient and potential liability.

Get Connected

1. Print the exposure control plan and review as a classroom discussion, reviewing the importance of its use when an exposure occurs.
2. Student should select and report certification requirements, including obtaining information about the testing process, the information or competencies included in the test, test application process, and continuing education requirements.

Glossary

A

accreditation The process by which a governmental agency evaluates a program or institution according to established guidelines or standards.

accuracy Achieving complete correctness or acceptable measures as close as possible to the true value.

additive Any substance such as an anticoagulant, antiglycolytic agent, separator gel, cell preservative, or clot activator added to a blood collection tube.

aerobic Any microorganism that can live and grow in the presence of oxygen or air.

aerosol Substances or particles suspended in a gas or the air.

agglutination The clumping of red blood cells that occurs from the binding of antibodies and antigens.

aliquoting Dividing or separating samples into separate containers.

American Certification Agency (ACA) National certification agency for health care professionals including phlebotomists and phlebotomy instructors.

American Medical Technologist (AMT) Organization that provides certification to phlebotomy personnel and approves phlebotomy programs.

American Society of Clinical Pathologists (ASCP) Agency responsible for providing clinical laboratory personnel certification, including phlebotomists.

American Society of Phlebotomy Technicians (ASPT) Professional organization for phlebotomists that also provides certification.

anaerobic Any microorganism that can live and grow in the absence of oxygen or air.

analyte A substance undergoing analysis, such as glucose or cholesterol.

antecubital fossa Area located in the middle of the arm, in front of the elbow, that houses veins most commonly used for venipuncture.

antibody Complex protein substance that is produced in the presence of foreign substances such as bacteria, viruses, lipids, or carbohydrates in order to protect the body.

anticoagulant Any agent that prevents blood from clotting.

antigen A substance that causes the formation of an antibody when introduced into blood or tissue.

antiglycolytic Glucose preservative found in some blood collection tubes.

antiseptic Germicidal solution used to clean the skin prior to venipuncture or dermal puncture.

aorta Largest artery in the body.

arteriole A smaller branch of an artery; a miniature artery.

artery A blood vessel that carries blood from the heart to the tissues.

aseptic Pertaining to a condition that is free of disease-producing microorganisms (germs).

assault An unlawful act of threatening or causing a person to experience fear.

assay A test, examination, or laboratory analysis of a substance.

atrium (atria, plural) One of two top chambers of the heart, known as the holding chambers.

autoantibody Immunoglobulin created in response to damaged antigens on the surface of one's own blood or body cells.

B

bacteremia The presence of bacteria in the blood.

bacteriostatic Substance that is capable of inhibiting the growth of bacteria.

basal state Metabolic condition after 12 hours of fasting and lack of exercise.

basilic vein Vein used for venipuncture that is not well anchored and tends to roll.

basophil Least numerous type of leukocytes; the granules are large and stain dark blue from basic dyes and often obscure the nucleus.

battery The unlawful use of physical force or contact toward another individual.

bedside manner Behavior that puts a patient at ease while health care personnel perform a procedure.

bevel Point of the needle that has been cut on a slant for ease of entry.

bleeding time The time it takes a standardized skin wound to stop bleeding; a test used to evaluate platelet function during clotting.

blood type A description based on the ABO classification system that determines the presence of specific antigens on the surface of red blood cells.

butterfly needle set Winged infusion set; used mostly for small veins or difficult venipuncture.

C

calcaneus The heel bone in the foot.

calibration Comparison of a known constant to the test equipment reading or measurement.

cannula A hollow tube used for temporary access to a vein or artery to administer medication or draw blood.

capillary The smallest of all blood vessels, which allow the exchange of nutrients and oxygen between the cells and blood; capillaries connect arteries to veins.

capillary action Process in which blood automatically flows into a thin tube.

capillary tube A disposable, small-diameter tube that fills by capillary action.

Centers for Disease Control and Prevention (CDC) Federal agency responsible for identifying, monitoring, and reporting diseases, especially infectious diseases capable of becoming widespread or epidemic.

centrifuge To spin blood samples at high speeds to separate the cellular portion from the liquid portion of blood; the instrument that performs this task.

centrifugation The process of separating the cells and plasma of blood using a device that spins the blood at high speeds, known as a centrifuge.

cephalic vein Vein used for venipuncture that may be difficult to palpate.

certification Process whereby individuals or institutions demonstrate their ability to perform at or above a predetermined level of standard.

chain of custody A special protocol that must be strictly followed and documented for specimen accountability.

chain of infection The six steps (links) that must take place for infection to occur (reservoir, infectious agent, portal of exit, mode of transmission, portal of entry, and susceptible host).

chemistry Evaluation of chemical constituents that normally occur in the human body, such as glucose, sodium, and potassium.

Clinical and Laboratory Standards Institute (CLSI) Nonprofit organization that sets recommendations, guidelines, or standards for all areas of the laboratory to improve the quality of medical care.

Clinical Laboratory Improvement Amendment (CLIA'88) Federal legislation that became effective in 1992. It mandates that all laboratories be regulated using the same standards, regardless of size, type, or location.

coagulation Cessation of bleeding; clot formation.

cold agglutinin An antibody present in certain disease conditions such as primary atypical pneumonia. These antibodies are located on the surface of the red blood cells, and at temperatures lower than normal body temperature they cause the blood cells to clump together.

collapsed vein An abnormal retraction of the vessel walls, stopping bloodflow.

concentric circles Circular motion starting from the center and moving outward in ever-widening even circles.

confidentiality Privacy regarding patient information.

control substance A substance or device used when doing equipment system checks.

culture media Material added to blood collection tubes that enhances the growth of microorganisms.

cytoplasm Area of the cell outside the Nucleus.

D

deoxygenated Presence of a larger quantity of carbon dioxide than oxygen.

dermal Pertaining to the skin.

dermal puncture Use of a sharp device to remove a small specimen of capillary blood.

diabetes mellitus Any of several related endocrine disorders characterized by an elevated level of glucose in the blood, caused by a deficiency of insulin or insulin resistance at the cellular level.

diapedesis Process by which certain white blood cells can exit the capillaries and enter the tissues in response to pathogens.

differential A hematology test that is a microscopic examination of a monolayer stained blood smear; indicates the percentage of different types of white blood cells, the number of both platelets and white blood cells, red blood cell size and shape, and any other blood abnormalities such as leukemia.

dilate To enlarge or increase the diameter.

disinfectant Solution that contains an agent intended to kill or irreversibly inactivate microorganisms.

distal phalanx Situated away from the center of the finger.

diurnal variation Normal changes in laboratory values throughout the day.

E

ecchymosis Discoloration or bruising caused by the seeping of blood underneath the skin.

edema A condition in which there is an accumulation of fluid in the tissues; usually resulting in swelling.

edematous Marked by edema, the result of swelling due to fluid accumulation.

eosinophil Leukocyte whose granules stain bright orange-red from eosin; aid the body in fighting parasites and are increased in allergies.

erythrocyte Red blood cell; an anuclear, biconcave disk blood cell that is responsible for transporting oxygen.

ethics An area of philosophy that examines values, actions, and choices to determine right and wrong.

evacuated collection tube Stoppered glass or plastic tube used for collecting blood that contains a premeasured vacuum.

evacuated tube holder Specialized plastic adaptor that holds both a needle and a tube for blood collection; *adaptor* or *barrel* are also common names.

F

false negative A test result that does not indicate a condition or substance that is actually present.

false positive A test result that indicates a positive result that is not true.

fasting Abstinence from food and liquids (except for water) for a specified period.

fibrin A filamentous protein formed by the action of thrombin on fibrinogen.

fibrinogen A protein found in plasma that is essential for clotting of blood.

G

gauge Unit of measure assigned to the diameter of the lumen (hole) of a needle.

gestational diabetes Elevated blood sugar during pregnancy.

glycolysis Normal body reaction in which glucose is hydrolyzed or broken down by an enzyme.

H

Health Insurance Portability and Accountability Act (HIPAA) A federal law that establishes a national standard for electronic health care transactions and protects the privacy and confidentiality of patient information. Among other provisions, HIPAA states that information about a patient must not be discussed with individuals other than the patient unless the patient has given written or verbal permission for you to do so.

hematocrit The percentage of space taken up by red blood cells in a whole blood sample; also referred to as *packed cell volume* and *microhematocrit*.

hematology Study of blood and blood-forming tissues.

hematoma Collection of blood under the skin due to leakage of blood from a punctured vein or artery.

hemochromatosis A disorder of iron metabolism in which too much iron is stored in the body, reaching toxic levels of iron.

hemoconcentration A rapid increase in the ratio of blood components (cells) to plasma (liquid).

hemoglobin Iron-rich protein molecules found in red blood cells that function to transport oxygen and carbon dioxide.

hemolysis Destruction of red blood cells that allows hemoglobin to be released from the red blood cell.

hemostasis The process of coagulation, or clot formation, that repairs vessel damage and stops blood loss.

hepatitis Inflammation of the liver from viral or toxic origin; can be caused by transmission through blood and body fluids.

histology Study of human body tissues and cells.

human immunodeficiency virus (HIV) Virus that causes acquired immune deficiency syndrome (AIDS).

I

immunology Study of how the body resists allergies and other agents that affect the body's immune system; also called *serology*.

informed consent Permission granted by the patient to perform any treatment; obtained only after the patient has been told what to expect, the risks, and usually the consequences of the procedure.

interstitial fluid The fluid present between cells and tissues.

isolation precautions Practices to prevent the spread of infection based upon how the infectious agent is transmitted.

K

keloid A sharply elevated, irregularly shaped, progressively enlarging scar formed by excessive collagen in the skin during healing.

L

leukocyte White blood cell; round cell with a nucleus whose main function is to combat infection and remove disintegrating tissues.

liability Legal obligation to compensate another for loss or damages.

lipemic Cloudy serum or plasma following or caused by increased lipids.

litigation Legal action or lawsuit.

lymphocyte A leukocyte produced in the lymphoid tissue; a nongranular leukocyte that has a role in the body's immune system.

lymphostasis Lack of fluid drainage in the lymph system, usually caused by lymph node removal.

M

malpractice Implies bad or dishonorable behavior.

Material safety data sheets (MSDS) Documentation of specific chemical ingredients found in hazardous substances, and emergency instructions to follow if abnormal contact occurs.

median cubital vein Most commonly used vein for venipuncture found in the middle of the forearm.

microbiology The study of one-cell organisms (microorganisms) that are usually visible only under a microscope; the main focus is bacteria.

microcollection The process of obtaining blood using a dermal (skin) puncture procedure, also known as *microtechnique*.

microhematocrit tube Type of capillary tube used for measuring a hematocrit, or packed cell volume.

microsample A sample of less than one milliliter.

microsurgery Surgery involving reconstruction of small tissue structures.

microtechnique Process of obtaining blood using a dermal (skin) puncture procedure; also known as *microcollection*.

monocyte A large leukocyte formed in bone marrow, with abundant cytoplasm and a kidney-shaped nucleus; function is to ingest bacteria and debris in tissues.

N

National Accrediting Agency for Clinical Laboratory Sciences (NAACLS) Organization that provides accreditation to phlebotomy training programs and offers certification for structured educational programs.

National Center for Competency Testing (NCCT) Independent third-party organization that provides certification testing for phlebotomy technicians.

National Credentialing Agency for Medical Laboratory Personnel (NCA) One of the agencies responsible for laboratory personnel certification.

National Healthcareer Association (NHA) Agency that provides certification and continuing education to health care professionals, including certified phlebotomy technicians.

negligence An intentional or unintentional error or wrongdoing.

neutrophil Leukocyte that engulfs and digests pathogens found in tissues; its granules stain lavender.

normal flora Microorganisms that typically live on and in the body, normally causing no harm to the host.

nosocomial infection Infection acquired while in a hospital or medical setting.

O

Occupational Safety and Health Administration (OSHA) A federal body responsible for preventing or minimizing employee injuries and exposure to harmful agents.

osteomyelitis Infection or inflammation of the bone or bone marrow.

outcome Results of a test or procedure.

oxygenated Containing a higher concentration of oxygen than carbon dioxide.

P

packed cell volume A synonym for hematocrit.

palmar Pertaining to the palm side of the hand.

palpable Detectable or noticeable by using touch; capable of being palpated.

palpate Examine by touching with the fingers, using pressure, then releasing.

Patient's Bill of Rights Document created by the American Hospital Association that identifies privileges health care facility patients are to have.

peak level Specimen collected when a serum drug level is at its highest level, usually 15 to 30 minutes after administration.

performance improvement Effort of all team members to improve the complete quality of the entire health care facility, not just of services requiring clinical skills; involves employees learning from their mistakes and from input of co-workers.

personal protective equipment (PPE) Protective coverings such as gloves, goggles, gowns, and masks that are worn to minimize exposure to blood and body fluids; required by OSHA to be worn when handling body fluids.

petechiae Small, nonraised red spots appearing on the skin due to minor hemorrhage in underlying tissue.

phagocytosis A process by which bacteria and antigens are surrounded and engulfed by leukocytes.

phlebotomist An individual trained and skilled in obtaining blood samples for clinical testing.

phlebotomy An invasive procedure in which a sharp object is introduced into a vein to obtain blood.

plantar Pertaining to the sole or bottom of the foot.

plasma The clear, pale yellow fluid component of blood that contains fibrinogen obtained from a tube that has an anticoagulant and has been centrifuged.

platelet function assay (PFA) Blood test that determines platelet adhesion and aggregation.

point-of-care testing (POCT) Tests performed at the patient's bedside or work area, using a portable instrument.

polycythemia A condition in which there is an overproduction of red blood cells.

postprandial After eating a meal.

pre-analytical error Error made before, during, or after the collection of blood and before the actual analysis.

process Actual procedure or duty that is to be done to the patient.

professionalism A group of characteristics or qualities that display a positive image or code of ethics.

pulmonary arteries Arteries that transport deoxygenated blood to the lungs.

pus A substance containing old leukocytes, pathogens, and other debris, created at the site of infection once the white blood cells undergo phagocytosis.

Q

quality assurance (QA) A program consisting of established policies and procedures that govern all activities of individual health care facilities.

quality control (QC) A component of quality assurance that examines each procedural step for accuracy.

quantity not sufficient (QNS) Specimen amount is too small to perform the ordered test.

R

reference laboratory An offsite lab to which specimens are referred for testing; usually used for tests not routinely performed in physicians' offices.

reference values Expected values for a laboratory or population, usually established using patients in a basal state.

reliable Believable and dependable.

requisition Form used to order a blood test, usually generated by or at the request of a physician.

Rh antigen A protein originally found on the red blood cells of the Rhesus monkey.

risk management A department in health care facilities that generates policies and procedures to protect patients, employees, and the employer from loss or injury.

S

sclerosis The abnormal hardening of tissue.

septicemia Presence of pathogenic microorganisms in the blood, causing symptoms such as fever, chills, and changes in mental state.

septum A muscular wall between the left and right side of the heart.

serology The identification of antibodies in the blood's serum.

serum Clear, pale yellow fluid that remains after blood clots and is separated; does not contain fibrinogen; plasma minus the clotting factors.

sphygmomanometer A device for measuring arterial blood pressure.

Standard Precautions Infection control guidelines issued by the CDC to decrease exposure to potentially infectious substances in acute care settings.

sterile Free of microorganisms.

supine Face upward, lying on the back.

syncope Fainting.

syringe Device that consists of a plunger and a barrel graduated in milliliters or cubic centimeters.

T

therapeutic drug monitoring Management of an effective drug dose by the physician.

therapeutic medication Relates to the treatment, remedy, or curing of a disorder through the use of a medicinal substance.

thrombin Enzyme formed in response to an injury that is a prerequisite to the fibrin clot formation.

thrombocyte Also called *platelet*; the smallest of the formed elements in the bloodstream.

total quality management (TQM) An institution-wide concept that involves all members of the health care team in creating quality processes to improve customer satisfaction.

tourniquet Device that impedes or stops the flow of blood.

toxicology Detection and study of agents that are harmful to the body.

trough level Specimen collected when a serum drug level is at its lowest level, usually immediately before the next scheduled dose is administered.

tunica adventitia Outermost covering of arteries and veins.

tunica intima Innermost layer of arteries and veins.

tunica media Middle layer of arteries and veins.

U

Unopette® A collection system designed for hematology tests, used to make accurate dilutions of whole blood.

urinalysis Examination of urine for physical, chemical, and microscopic characteristics.

V

vein Blood vessel that transports blood from body tissues back to the heart.

vena cava The largest vein in the body.

venipuncture Procedure in which a sharp object is introduced into a vein for the purpose of withdrawing blood or instilling medications.

venous reflux The backward flow of blood into the patient's veins during venipuncture.

ventricle (ventricles, plural) One of two bottom chambers of the heart known as the pumping chambers.

venule A minute vein.

W

waived tests Laboratory tests approved by the FDA that are minimally complicated and pose little risk of harm to the patient.

winged set Also called a *butterfly needle set*; consists of a stainless steel collection needle connected to 5 to 12 inches of plastic tubing.

Credits

Chapter 1

1.2 (*both*): © Total Care Programming, Inc.; **1.4:** © Vol. 72/PhotoDisc/Getty Images; **1.5:** © Total Care Programming, Inc.; **1.6 (*left*):** © The McGraw-Hill Companies, Inc./Jill Braaten, photographer; **1.6 (*right*):** Photo courtesy of STERIS Corporation, Mentor, Ohio, © 2007; **1.8a-c:** © The McGraw-Hill Companies, Inc./Jan L. Saeger, photographer.

Chapter 2

2.11b: © Bill Longcore/Photo Researchers, Inc.; **p. 46 (*all*):** © Ed Reschke.

Chapter 3

3.2: Requisition screen taken from LabDAQ® Laboratory Information System, courtesy of Antek-HealthWare, LLC. **3.3:** © Total Care Programming, Inc.; **3.4:** © Stockbyte/Punchstock; **3.5a-b, 3.6a-b:** © Total Care Programming, Inc.; **p. 70 (*all*), 3.8a-c:** Courtesy and © Becton Dickinson; **3.10a-b:** © Total Care Programming, Inc.; **3 14:** Courtesy and © Becton Dickinson; **3.15 (*left*):** © Total Care Programming, Inc.; **3.15 (*right-both*):** Courtesy and © Becton Dickinson; **3.16:** © Total Care Programming, Inc.; **3.17:** © Terry Wild Studios.

Chapter 4

4.1: © Total Care Programming, Inc.; **4.2:** © David M. Grossman/Phototake; **4.3, 4.5, 4.6, 4.8, 4.10a-b, 4.11, 4.15-4.23, 4.26, 4.29:** © Total Care Programming, Inc.; **4.14:** Courtesy of Venoscope, LLC.

Chapter 5

5.1, 5.2, 5.6a-c, 5.7, 5.8a-b, 5.10, 5.11a-c, 5.12, 5.14, 5.15: © Total Care Programming, Inc.

Chapter 6

6.1, 6.2, 6.3: © Clinical Chemistry, QEII Health Sciences Centre, Halifax, Nova Scotia, Canada; **6.4:** © Yoav Levy/Phototake; **6.5:** © Antonio Reeve/Photo Researchers; **6.6:** Courtesy of Tri-Tech, Inc.; **6.7:** © Total Care Programming, Inc.

Index

Blood cultures, 67, 119
Blood pressure cuff
        (sphygmomanometer), 167
Blood smear procedure, 49, 146–149
Blood thinners (heparin and warfarin)
        and therapeutic drug monitoring
        (TDM), 47, 52, 183
Blood-borne pathogens, 17–18
Bloodletting, 2–3
Bone infection, osteomyelitis, 125
Buffy coat, 49
Butterfly needle set, 120–122
    collecting blood culture specimens,
        142–143
    and safe-needle devices, 70
    using for veins on back of hand, 104

C

Calcaneus, 125
Calibration and control check of
        equipment, 198–200
Cannula, 184
Capillaries, 33–36, 39
Capillary action, 6–7, 81–83
    capillary tubes, 148–149
    microcollection, 127–128, 146–150
Carbon dioxide partial pressure, 185
Cardiac enzymes, 167
Centers for Disease Control and
        Prevention (CDC), 13, 17–18,
        24, 29
Central venous therapy lines, 185
Centrifugation, centrifuged blood
        sample, 49, 93
    centrifuge operation, 159–160
    microhematocrit centrifuge,
        149–150
Cephalic vein, 40, 41, 100
Certificate of Waiver, 154
Certification for phlebotomists, 6,
        193–194
Chain of custody, 22, 23, 143, 167,
        180–182
    laboratory form for (sample), 144
    legal specimens, 143, 179–180
Chain of infection, 15–16
Chemistry, 10
Children
    dermal puncture, 81, 119–125
    and elderly patients with fragile veins
        and skin, 80
        special considerations for
            bandaging, 116, 129
        special considerations for
            venipuncture, 104–106
    glucose testing, 171
Chilled and light-sensitive specimen
        collection, 145, 200
Chlorhexidene gluconate, 67
Choking, prevention of, 102,
        116, 129
Chordae tendineae, 32
Circles, concentric, cleansing puncture
        site, 106
Citrate phosphate dextrose
        (CPD-A1), 177

Cleansing puncture site
    blood culture site cleaning procedure,
        141–142
    nonalcohol cleansers required,
        180, 181
    venipuncture site, 106, 107
Clinical and Laboratory Standards
        Institute (CLSI), 2, 13, 193
Clinical Laboratory Improvement Act
        (CLIA '88), 11, 13
Clinical Laboratory Improvement
        Advisory Committee
        (CLIAC), 154
Clotting factors, 51–52
Coagulation, 49, 50
Coban® bandage, 68, 116
Cold agglutinins, testing for, 143, 145
Collagen fibers, 51
Collapsed vein, 116
College of American Pathologists (CAP),
        13, 29
Color coding of evacuated tubes, 75,
        76–78
Communication and customer
        service, 7–9
    do not discuss test with patient, 113
    geriatric patients (elderly), 105
    patients unable to communicate, 8,
        92–94
    pediatric patients (children), 105, 106
    preventing allergies and bleeding, 69
Computers in the laboratory, 63–64
Confidentiality of information and
        patients' privacy, 20–21
Consent, informed, written, and
        implied, 22
    patient's refusal, 23, 97, 173
Contact transmission, infection, 16
Continuing education for
        phlebotomists, 194
Control substance and calibration,
        198–200
Coronary arteries and circulation, 32
Cortisol levels, 167
Coumadin, 52
Cross-training, 203
Culture media, 138, 143
Cupping, 3
Cytoplasm of white blood cells, 45, 46

D

Department of Health and Human
        Services (DHHS), 13
Dermal puncture, 2, 6, 7
    collection devices, 81–83, 121–123
    fingerprints, 127
    performing a dermal puncture, 123–129
    warming puncture site, 81–82, 125
Diabetes, 170
Diapedesis, 45
Dietary restrictions, verifying, 96
Differential blood test, 47, 151
Direct Coombs blood test, 54
Discrimination against patients, 21–22
Disinfectant, 180
Diurnal variation, 167, 197

Documentation
    equipment quality checks, 200
    of errors, 196–197
    of exposure incident, 203, 204
    medicolegal, 127, 143, 179–182
    of patient's status, 95–96
    to prevent liability, 203
    of problems, 23, 93, 97
    of specimens not collected, 93
    of tests, 200
Dorsal venous arch, 41
Dress code and professional
        appearance, 7
Droplet infection transmission, 16
Drugs, therapeutic monitoring (TDM),
        115, 176–177

E

Ecchymoses, 112
Edema, 95, 104, 126
Education, continuing, for
        phlebotomists, 194
Elderly patients and children with fragile
        veins, 79–81
    special considerations for
        venipuncture, 104–106
Employment locations for phlebotomists,
        10, 24
Enzymes, cardiac, 167
Eosinophils, 45, 46, 47
Equipment, calibration and control
        check, 198–200
Errors
    air bubbles, 82, 144
    arterial puncture, accidental, 39
    avoiding accidents, 39, 40
    dermal puncture, 125, 127
    documentation of, 196–197
    factors affecting laboratory values,
        200, 207
    median nerve, avoid during
        venipuncture, 40
    needlestick injuries, 18, 71
    pre-analytical error, 138
Erythroblastosis fetalis, 54
Erythrocyte Sedimentation Rate (ESR),
        117, 123
Erythrocytes (red blood cells), 42, 43–44
Escherichia coli, 140
Ethical responsibility and redraw of
        specimen, 201
Evacuated tubes and tube holders,
        71, 72, 73–74
    antiglycolytic, glucose preservative
        agent, 78
    color coding of evacuated tubes,
        75, 76–78
Evaluation of processes, outcomes,
        196–197
Eye protection, 18, 19, 154

F

Face shield, 18, 19, 154
Factors and variables affecting test
        results and values, 168, 200, 207